Your *Clinics* subscription just got better!

You can now access the FULL TEXT of this publication online at no additional cost! Activate your online subscription today and receive...

- Full text of all issues from 2002 to the present
- Photographs, tables, illustrations, and references
- Comprehensive search capabilities
- Links to MEDLINE and Elsevier journals

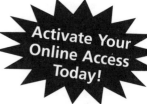

Plus, you can also sign up for E-alerts of upcoming issues or articles that interest you, and take advantage of exclusive access to bonus features!

To activate your individual online subscription:

1. Visit our website at **www.TheClinics.com**.

2. Click on "Register" at the top of the page, and follow the instructions.

3. To activate your account, you will need your subscriber account number, which you can find on your mailing label (note: the number of digits in your subscriber account number varies from six to ten digits). See the sample below where the subscriber account number has been circled.

This is your subscriber account number

```
************************************************3-DIGIT 001
FEB00   J0167   C7   (123456-89)   10/00   Q: 1

J.H. DOE, MD
531 MAIN ST
CENTER CITY, NY  10001-001
```

4. That's it! Your online access to the most trusted source for clinical reviews is now available.

theclinics.com

ELSEVIER

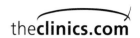

FOOT AND ANKLE CLINICS

Achilles Tendon

GUEST EDITOR
Nicola Maffulli, MD, MS, PhD, FRCS(Orth)

CONSULTING EDITOR
Mark S. Myerson, MD

June 2005 • Volume 10 • Number 2

SAUNDERS

An Imprint of Elsevier, Inc.
PHILADELPHIA   LONDON   TORONTO   MONTREAL   SYDNEY   TOKYO

W.B. SAUNDERS COMPANY
A Division of Elsevier Inc.

1600 John F. Kennedy Blvd., Suite 1800, Philadelphia, PA 19103-2899

http://www.theclinics.com

FOOT AND ANKLE CLINICS　　　　　　　　　　　　　　　　　**Volume 10, Number 2**
June 2005　　　　　　　　　　　　　　　　　　　　　　　　**ISSN 1083-7515**
Editor: Debora Dellapena　　　　　　　　　　　　　　　　　**ISBN 1-4160-2655-X**

Foot and Ankle Clinics (ISSN 1083-7515) is published quarterly by Elsevier; Corporate and editorial Offices: 1600 John F. Kennedy Blvd., Suite 1800, Philadelphia, PA 19103-2899. Accounting and circulation offices: 6277 Sea Harbor Drive, Orlando, FL 32887-4800. Periodicals postage paid at Orlando, FL 32862, and additional mailing offices. Subscription prices are $160.00 per year for US individuals, $232.00 per year for US institutions, $80.00 per year for US students and residents, $180.00 per year for Canadian individuals, $269.00 per year for Canadian institutions, $210.00 for international individuals, $269.00 for international institutions and $105.00 per year for Canadian and foreign students residents. To receive student/resident rate, orders must be accompanied by name of affiliated institution, date of term, and the *signature* of program/residency coordinator on institution letterhead. Orders will be billed at individual rate until proof of status is received. Foreign air speed delivery is included in all *Clinics* subscription prices. All prices are subject to change without notice. POSTMASTER: Send address changes to *Foot and Ankle Clinics*, W.B. Saunders Company, Periodicals Fulfillment, Orlando, FL 32887-4800. **Customer Service: 1-800-654-2452 (US). From outside of the US, call 1-407-345-1000.**

Printed in the United States of America.

CONSULTING EDITOR

MARK S. MYERSON, MD, President, American Orthopedic Foot and Ankle Society; Director, Institute for Foot and Ankle Reconstruction, Mercy Medical Center, Baltimore, Maryland

GUEST EDITOR

NICOLA MAFFULLI, MD, MS, PhD, FRCS(Orth), Professor, Department of Trauma and Orthopaedic Surgery, Keele University School of Medicine, Staffordshire, United Kingdom

CONTRIBUTORS

HÅKAN ALFREDSON, MD, PhD, Professor, Sports Medicine Unit, Department of Surgical and Perioperative Science, Umeå University, Umeå, Sweden

ROBERT R. BLEAKNEY, MB, BCH, MRAD, FRCR, Assistant Professor, Joint Department of Medical Imaging, University Health Network and Mount Sinai Hospitals, University of Toronto, Toronto, Ontario, Canada

W.H.B. EDWARDS, MB, BS, Dip Anat, MS, FRACS (Orth), FAOrthA, Surgeon, Orthopaedic Foot and Ankle Centre of Victoria, Victoria, Australia

TERO A.H. JÄRVINEN, MD, PhD, Assistant Professor, Department of Orthopaedic Surgery, Tampere University Hospital; Medical School and the Institute of Medical Technology, University of Tampere, Tampere, Finland; The Burnham Institute, La Jolla, California

PEKKA KANNUS, MD, PhD, Professor, Chief Physician, Department of Orthopaedic Surgery, Tampere University Hospital; Medical School and the Institute of Medical Technology, University of Tampere; Accident and Trauma Research Center and the Tampere Research Center of Sports Medicine, UKK Institute, Tampere, Finland

KARIM M. KHAN, MD, PhD, Assistant Professor, Department of Family Practice (Sports Medicine) and School of Human Kinetics, University of British Columbia, Vancouver, British Columbia, Canada

SHEKHAR M. KUMTA, MD, PhD, Department of Orthopaedics and Traumatology, The Chinese University of Hong Kong, Prince of Wales Hospital, Shatin, Hong Kong

HAMISH D.H. LESLIE, MB, ChB, FRACS, Fellow, Orthopaedic Foot and Ankle Centre of Victoria, Victoria, Australia

NICOLA MAFFULLI, MD, MS, PhD, FRCS(Orth), Professor, Department of Trauma and Orthopaedic Surgery, Keele University School of Medicine, Staffordshire, United Kingdom

MERZESH MAGRA, MRCS, Research Fellow, Department of Trauma and Orthopaedic Surgery, Keele University School of Medicine, Staffordshire, United Kingdom

DONALD J. McBRIDE, FRCS(Orth), Department of Trauma and Orthopaedics, Keele University School of Medicine, Hartshill, United Kingdom

TOMAS MOVIN, MD, PhD, Department of Orthopedics, Huddinge Hospital, Karolinska Institute, Stockholm, Sweden

MARK S. MYERSON, MD, President, American Orthopedic Foot and Ankle Society; Director, Institute for Foot and Ankle Reconstruction, Mercy Medical Center, Baltimore, Maryland

MOIRA O'BRIEN, FRCPI, FFSEMI, Professor, Department of Anatomy, Trinity College, University of Dublin, Dublin, Ireland

FRANCESCO OLIVA, MD, Department of Trauma and Orthopaedic Surgery, Keele University School of Medicine, North Staffordshire Hospital, Staffordshire, United Kingdom

MIKA PAAVOLA, MD, PhD, Department of Orthopaedics and Traumatology, Helsinki University Central Hospital; Department of Orthopaedics and Traumatology, Töölö Hospital, Helsinki, Finland; Medical School and the Institute of Medical Technology, University of Tampere, Tampere, Finland

ÅSA RYBERG, MD, Department of Orthopedic Surgery, Karolinska Institute, Centre for Surgical Studies, Karolinska University Hospital/Huddinge, Stockholm, Sweden

MURALI KRISHNA SAYANA, MBBS, MS, AFRCSI, Department of Trauma and Orthopaedic Surgery, Keele University School of Medicine, Staffordshire, United Kingdom

PANKAJ SHARMA, MBBS, MRCS, Department of Trauma and Orthopaedic Surgery, Wessex Deanery, United Kingdom; Department of Trauma and Orthopaedics, Keele University School of Medicine, United Kingdom

ANAND M. VORA, MD, Lake Forest Orthopaedic Associates, Illinois Bone and Joint Institute Ltd., Libertyville, Illinois

LAWRENCE M. WHITE, MD, FRCP(C), Associate Professor and Head, Division of Musculoskeletal Imaging, Joint Department of Medical Imaging, University Health Network and Mount Sinai Hospitals, University of Toronto, Toronto, Ontario, Canada

JONATHAN S. YOUNG, MRCS, Department of Trauma and Orthopaedic Surgery, Keele University School of Medicine, North Staffordshire Hospital, Staffordshire, United Kingdom

CONTENTS

> The Achilles tendon is the strongest and largest tendon in the body.
> It is the conjoined tendon of the gastrocnemius and the soleus mus-
> cles, and may have a small contribution from the plantaris. The
> muscles and the Achilles tendon are in the posterior, superficial
> compartment of the calf. Through the Achilles tendon, they are the
> main plantar flexors of the ankle. The Achilles tendon is subjected
> to the highest loads in the body, with tensile loads up to ten times
> body weight during running, jumping, hopping, and skipping.
> This article discusses the anatomy of the Achilles tendon.

> The Achilles tendon is the most commonly injured tendon in the
> foot and ankle; injuries commonly are related to sports/athletic
> activities. Imaging modalities that are used most commonly in the
> diagnostic assessment of the Achilles tendon include conventional
> radiography, ultrasonography, and MRI. This article reviews the
> normal and pathologic imaging features of the Achilles tendon, and
> highlights the potential usefulness and limitations of various imag-
> ing techniques in the noninvasive assessment of the tendon and the
> potential impact of imaging findings on clinical patient care.

Achilles Tendon Disorders: Etiology and Epidemiology

Tero A.H. Järvinen, Pekka Kannus, Nicola Maffulli, and Karim M. Khan

The Achilles tendon is the strongest tendon in the human body. Because most Achilles tendon injuries take place in sports and there has been a general increase in popularity of sporting activities, the number and incidence of the Achilles tendon overuse injuries and complete, spontaneous ruptures has increased in the industrialized countries during the last decades. The most common clinical diagnosis of Achilles overuse injuries is tendinopathy. The basic etiology of the Achilles tendinopathy is known to be multifactorial. Although histopathologic studies have shown that ruptured Achilles tendons have clear degenerative changes before the rupture, many Achilles tendon ruptures take place suddenly without any preceding signs or symptoms.

Molecular Events in Tendinopathy: A Role for Metalloproteases

Merzesh Magra and Nicola Maffulli

Disorganized, haphazard ineffective healing is a constant feature of chronic tendinopathy. Normal tendon is composed mostly of type I collagen. Tendinopathic tendons, conversely, have a greater proportion of type III collagen, which is associated with tendon rupture. Matrix metalloproteinases (MMPs) are involved in remodelling of the extracellular matrix (ECM) of tendons, because they are either up- or down-regulated in tendinopathy. A balance between MMPs and tissue inhibitors of metalloproteinases is required to maintain tendon homeostasis. The mechanism of activation of MMPs is poorly understood, and their precise role in tendinopathy is unclear.

Paratendinopathy

Mika Paavola and Tero A.H. Järvinen

Because most Achilles tendon injuries take place in sports and there has been a general increase in the popularity of sporting activities, the number and incidence of Achilles tendon overuse injuries have increased in the industrialized countries during the last few decades. The term "Achilles paratendinopathy" is used in clinical practice to describe activity-related Achilles pain combined with tenderness on palpation, providing that there is no suspicion of intratendinous pathology on the basis of patient history, clinical examination, or imaging examinations. This article discusses Achilles paratendinopathy.

anesthesia and followed by early functional rehabilitation are becoming increasingly common, and should be considered when managing such patients.

FORTHCOMING ISSUES

RECENT ISSUES

THE CLINICS ARE NOW AVAILABLE ONLINE!

http://www.theclinics.com

FOOT AND ANKLE CLINICS

Foot Ankle Clin N Am
10 (2005) xi–xii

Foreword

Achilles Tendon

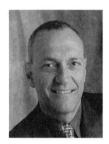

Mark S. Myerson, MD
Consulting Editor

This is an issue of which to be proud. Dr Nicola Maffulli has done a superb job of bringing together the world's leading authorities on problems of the Achilles tendon. I have found each manuscript in this issue to be exciting, innovative, and informative; these will set the standard for the management of diagnosis and treatment of rupture and tendinopathy for years to come.

It is amazing how much this field has advanced in the past decade. I recall the controversies of the early 1980s—whether to operate on the Achilles, how to treat an acute rupture, how best to use and to preserve autogenous tissue, how to prevent progression of tendinosis. Even the nomenclature has changed and fortunately so. For too long we have used incorrect terminology when describing Achilles tendon "dysfunction"; it is hoped that, for the foreseeable future, we can discontinue the use of the term "tendinitis" because there is no inflammatory component associated with these tendon disorders.

From a clinical perspective, our goal of treatment for most patients who have ruptures of the Achilles is to return them to their level of daily, athletic, and competitive activity as soon as possible, and with a minimum of complications. Certainly, the modified percutaneous techniques have accomplished these goals, and with early and aggressive rehabilitation, maximization of function is possible. Although nonoperative therapies are available for the management of acute ruptures, my personal bias, backed by clinical experience, has been the contrary; timely surgery using a modified percutaneous method with the

1083-7515/05/$ – see front matter © 2005 Elsevier Inc. All rights reserved.
doi:10.1016/j.fcl.2005.01.014

Achillon system has proven successful. Perhaps the greatest changes in diagnosis and treatment have come about in the management of tendinopathy, and this issue is replete with superb manuscripts that highlight current treatment concepts. My congratulations to all of the authors.

Mark S. Myerson, MD
Institute for Foot and Ankle Reconstruction
Mercy Medical Center
301 St. Paul Place
Baltimore MD 21202, USA
E-mail address: mark4feet@aol.com

ELSEVIER
SAUNDERS

Foot Ankle Clin N Am
10 (2005) xiii

FOOT AND
ANKLE CLINICS

Preface

Achilles Tendon

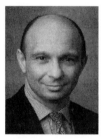

Nicola Maffulli, MD, MS, PhD, FRCS(Orth)
Guest Editor

The amount of clinical and basic science work that is performed on the Achilles tendon is phenomenal; nevertheless, we still lack many evidence-based practice guidelines. Some investigators are sanguine about their views, whereas others keep an open mind and continue to perform hypothesis-testing–based studies.

The Achilles tendon is subjected to overuse and acute injuries. We have managed to get together an international team that spans the Old and the New World to tackle a variety of issues on the Achilles tendon, ranging from the gross anatomy to the more sophisticated vision of the future, including gene therapy and tissue engineering.

As a guest editor, I have been blessed with a great writing team: to them my thanks. I hope that you will enjoy reading this issue as much as I enjoyed editing it.

Nicola Maffulli, MD, MS, PhD, FRCS(Orth)
Department of Trauma and Orthopaedic Surgery
Keele University School of Medicine
Thornburrow Drive
Hartshill, Stoke-on-Trent
Staffordshire ST4 7QB, UK
E-mail address: n.maffulli@keele.ac.uk

ELSEVIER
SAUNDERS

Foot Ankle Clin N Am
10 (2005) 225–238

FOOT AND
ANKLE CLINICS

The Anatomy of the Achilles Tendon

Moira O'Brien, FRCPI, FFSEMI

Department of Anatomy, Trinity College, University of Dublin, Dublin 2, Ireland

The Achilles tendon is the strongest and largest tendon in the body. It is the conjoined tendon of the gastrocnemius and the soleus muscles, and may have a small contribution from the plantaris. The muscles and the Achilles tendon are in the posterior, superficial compartment of the calf. Through the Achilles tendon, they are the main plantar flexors of the ankle. Fascial septa divide the posterior compartment into the superficial, deep, and deepest compartments [1,2]. The posterior compartment contains the plantar flexors of the ankle. The tibial nerve and the posterior tibial artery, the peroneal arteries, and their branches supply them.

The Achilles tendon is subjected to the highest loads in the body, with tensile loads up to ten times body weight during running, jumping, hopping, and skipping [3–7]. The Achilles tendon is subjected to stress when running up and down hill, particularly if there are associated biomechanical malalignments. A tight Achilles tendon also limits dorsiflexion of the ankle [8–10].

Recurrent Achilles tendon pain may be due to spondolysthesis at L5/S1 [11–15]. Achilles injuries occur annually in 7% to 9% of top class runners [7], and basketball, volleyball, and squash players [16,17].

The medial and lateral heads of the gastrocnemius with the plantaris cross the knee joint. When the knee is extended and the ankle is dorsiflexed, the gastrocnemius is stretched [19]. The gastrocnemius consists mainly of fast twitch fibers. It plantar flexes the foot on the ankle, propels the body forward, and flexes the knee. The soleus muscle originates below the knee, and therefore, has no action on the knee joint. The soleus is a postural muscle that is composed

---

E-mail address: mobrien@tcd.ie

1083-7515/05/$ – see front matter © 2005 Elsevier Inc. All rights reserved.
doi:10.1016/j.fcl.2005.01.011

mainly of slow twitch type I fibers. It also acts as a peripheral vascular pump [18,19].

Gastrocnemius

The gastrocnemius is the most superficial muscle. A fusiform muscle, it forms the lower boundary of the popliteal fossa and accounts for the bulge of the calf (Fig. 1) [2,20]. The medial head of the gastrocnemius arises from the popliteal surface of the femur behind the medial supracondylar line and the adductor tubercle, above the medial femoral condyle. It is larger and longer, and extends more distally in the calf than the lateral head [2].

The lateral head is shorter and arises from the posterior part of the lateral surface of the lateral femoral condyle, above and behind the lateral epicondyle and from a portion of the lateral lip of the linea aspera above the condyle. Both heads also arise from the oblique popliteal ligament—part of the capsule of the knee joint—and are attached to the condyles of the femur by strong flat tendons, which extend for a short distance on the posterior or the superficial surface of the muscles as an aponeurosis (Fig. 2) [21].

A sesamoid bone (the fabella) may be present in the lateral head at the point of maximum stress in 27% to 29% of individuals [21], and may give rise to the fabello-fibular ligament on the posterolateral portion of the capsule of the knee joint [22]. Bursae may lie deep to the two heads. The bursa deep to the medial head sometime communicates with the knee joint, and may be involved in Baker's cysts. The deep surface of the gastrocnemius, related to the soleus, is tendinous. The muscle bellies extend to the middle of the calf and as the two bellies of the gastrocnemius come together, they form a tendinous raphe that

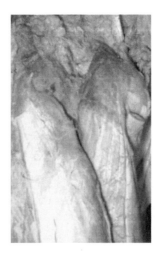

Fig. 1. Left medial and lateral heads of gastrocnemius, lower boundary of popliteal fossa.

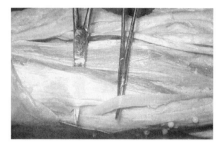

Fig. 2. Lateral head of gastrocnemius and common peroneal nerve under forceps.

becomes continuous with the aponeurosis on the anterior or deep aspect of the muscle. This unites with the tendon of the soleus to form the Achilles tendon (Fig. 3).

Soleus

The soleus muscle is a broad, flat pennate muscle. It is wider than the gastrocnemius, and its muscle fibers extend more distally than those of the gastrocnemius. It originates from the posterior surface of the head and upper

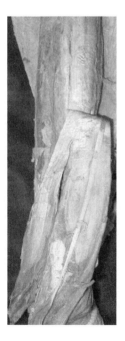

Fig. 3. Soleus and plantaris.

fourth of the posterior surface of the fibula, from a fibrous arch between fibula and tibia, and from the oblique line and the middle third of the medial border of the tibia. The popliteal vessels and the tibial nerve pass under the fibrous arch.

The soleus consists of two aponeurotic lamellae with the bulk of the vascular multi-pennate muscle fibers in between. The muscular fibers end in the posterior aponeurosis of the soleus, which lies anterior to the aponeurosis of the gastrocnemius. The aponeurotic fibers of the muscles lie parallel to each other for a variable distance before they unite [21]. Perforating veins from the great saphenous vein enter the soleus, which contains a rich plexus of veins. The soleus fuses with the gastrocnemius and forms the deepest portion of the Achilles tendon.

The tendinous portion of the soleus usually is the largest of the tendons that contribute to the Achilles tendon, and is the prime plantar flexor [16,17]. It is a postural muscle and keeps the body upright during standing. As the center of gravity passes in front of the axis of movement of the knee joint, the soleus contracts to counteract the tendency for the body to tilt forward at the ankle. It acts only on the ankle joint [19].

Two main types of anomalous soleus muscle can be recognized. The first is an extension of the muscle more distally than usual along the Achilles tendon. The second is a separate insertion of the soleus into the upper surface of the calcaneus with a separate tendon, or directly without a tendon. An anomalous soleus is found in less than 2% of patients who require Achilles surgery (Fig. 4) [14].

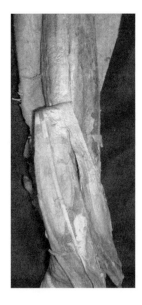

Fig. 4. Soleus, plantaris tendon lying on reflected posterior aspect of gastrocnemius.

Plantaris

The plantaris muscle has a variable size, and is absent in 6% to 8% of individuals. It has a short, fleshy origin from the popliteal surface of the femur above the lateral femoral condyle. The muscle belly is usually 5 cm to 10 cm in length, with a long tendon that extends distally between the gastrocnemius and the soleus. The tendon inserts into the medial border of the Achilles tendon, anterior to the Achilles tendon. In 6% to 8% of subjects, it inserts into the flexor retinaculum [21]. This tendon may rupture, and may be used as a tendon graft.

Achilles tendon

The Achilles tendon is approximately 15 cm long, and starts at the musculo-tendinous junction of the gastrocnemius and soleus in the middle of the calf. The tendon is flattened at its junction with the gastrocnemius to become rounded until approximately 4 cm from its insertion. At this level, it flattens, then ex-pands and becomes cartilaginous, to insert into a rough area on the middle of the lower part of the posterior surface of the calcaneus. On its anterior surface, it receives the muscular fibers from the soleus almost to its insertion (Fig. 5) [23,24].

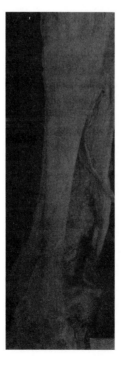

Fig. 5. Left Achilles tendon.

The soleus and the gastrocnemius vary in their orientation, contribution to the Achilles tendon, and the extent of their fusion [25]. In 52% of subjects, the soleus contributed 52% to the Achilles tendon, and the gastrocnemius contributed 48%. The fibers of the soleus formed the anterior and medial portion of the tendon. In 35% of subjects, the gastrocnemius and the soleus muscles contributed 50% each. In 13% of subjects, the gastrocnemius formed two thirds of the tendon. The tendinous portion of the soleus varies from 3 cm to 11 cm, and the gastrocnemius portion varies from 11 cm to 16 cm (Fig. 6) [24].

The tendon fibers spiral so that fibers that originate from the tibial side of the muscular mass pass obliquely from the deep to the superficial aspect, across the superficial surface of the tendon, to the lateral side. Fibers from the fibular side pass on the deep side of the tendon, to the tibial side of the insertion of the tendon [26]. As the Achilles tendon descends, it twists through 90°, and the gastrocnemius component is found mainly on the lateral and posterior part of the tendon. Some individuals exhibit a double spiral: the lateral head runs from the dorsal side, then comes ventral, and finally turns to the dorsal aspect. Rotation begins above the region where the soleus tends to join the gastrocnemius component, and the degree of rotation is greater if there is minimal fusion. Twisting produces an area of stress within the tendon, which is most marked 2 cm to 5 cm above its calcaneal insertion [27,28], is an area of poor vascularity, and is a common site of tendinopathy and rupture (Fig. 7) [14].

The insertion becomes broad distally and has a wide deltoid type of attachment, which varies from 1.2 cm to 2.5 cm [10]. The deep surface of the inferior portion of the tendon above its attachment to the calcaneus has an area of fibro-

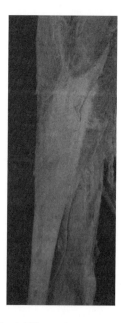

Fig. 6. Right Achilles tendon, medial head longer.

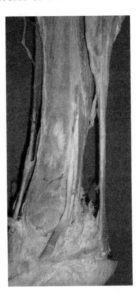

Fig. 7. Medial view of right Achilles insertion.

cartilage between the tendon and the upper part of calcaneus, where there is a similar area of fibro-cartilage [26,27].

Deep and just proximal to the insertion is the retrocalcaneal bursa, which lies between the tuberosity on the posterior surface of the calcaneus and the Achilles tendon. The bursa that is present at birth is a thick-walled, wedge-shaped sac. It has a horseshoe shape on cross-section; the arms extend distally on the medial and lateral edges of the tendon, with an average length of 22 mm, a width of 4 mm, and a depth of 8 mm [8]. The area of fibro-cartilage on the tendon forms the posterior wall. The anterior wall of the retrocalcaneal bursa is the 0.5-mm to 1-mm thick cartilaginous layer on the posterior aspect of the calcaneus. The proximal wall of the synovial-lined sac consists of folds, or villus synovial projections to allow alterations in its form, that are produced by varying degrees of pressure on the fat above it during flexion and extension of the ankle (M. Benjamin, personal communication) (Fig. 8) [29–31].

The area between the Achilles tendon, the posterior tibia, and the upper part of the posterior surface of the calcaneus is known as Karger's triangle, and separates the Achilles tendon from the deep flexors. The flexor hallucis longus lies below the fascial septum and the tibia. Blood vessels lie in Karger's triangle, and supply the Achilles tendon (Fig. 9) [8,26].

Some of the collagen fibers at the insertion of the tendon form Sharpey's fibers. The endotenon becomes continuous with the periosteum. There is no periosteum at the insertion [16,17], but some of the superficial fibers become continuous with fibrous tissue of the calcaneus and pass from the lower border of the calcaneus to join the plantar fascia [26,30]. The number of fibers that connect the Achilles tendon to the plantar fascia decreases with age.

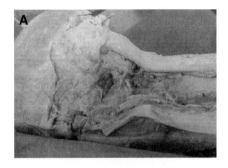

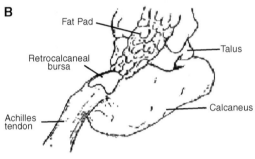

Fig. 8. (*A*) Achilles tendon and fat in Karger's triangle. (*B*) Retrocalcaneal bursa.

The superior tuberosity of the calcaneus can be hyperconcave, normal, or hypoconvex [8]. Haglund's bony deformity is an abnormal prominence on the posterosuperior lateral aspect of the calcaneus [8]. A superficial subcutaneous bursa lies between the skin and the Achilles tendon, and develops following chronic irritation and external compression from shoes.

Although there is no true synovial sheath around the Achilles tendon, it is enclosed by a paratenon, a thin gliding membrane of loose areolar tissue that is rich in mucopolysaccharides, continuous proximally with the fascial envelope of muscle, and blends distally with the periosteum of the calcaneus [32].The outermost layer is composed of loose, fatty areolar tissue, a loose fibrillar tissue

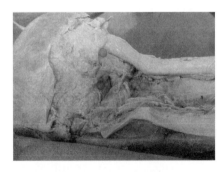

Fig. 9. Achilles tendon and fat in Karger's triangle.

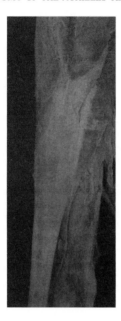

Fig. 10. Right Achilles tendon, medial head longer.

that functions as an elastic tissue and allows a wide range of movement [33]. Its mechanical function is to allow the tendon to glide freely against the surrounding tissue. The connective tissue that surrounds the fibrils, fascicles, and the entire muscle consists mainly of type I collagen with a minor component that consists of type III collagen. Type IV collagen is found in the basement membrane, as are traces of type V collagen. Nerves and blood vessels run through the paratenon. Fluid may be found between the paratenon and the epitenon and prevents friction (Fig. 10) [34].

Structure of the Achilles tendon

Tendons appear white because they are mostly avascular. A tendon is a roughly uniaxial composite that is composed of mainly type I collagen in an extracellular matrix that is composed of mucopolysaccharide and a proteoglycan gel [35]. They consist of 30% collagen and 2% elastin embedded in an extracellular matrix that contains 68% water and tenocytes [36,37]. Elastin contributes to the flexibility of the tendon. The collagen protein, tropocollagen, forms 65% to 80% of the mass of dry weight tendons.

The Achilles tendon consists of typical parallel bundles of type I collagen (tropocollagen). The average size of the collagen fibers of the Achilles tendon is 60 μm. Collagen fibrils in the Achilles vary from 30 nm to 130 nm in diameter, although most are between 50 nm and 90 nm in diameter. Collagen forms

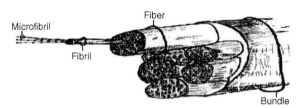

Fig. 11. The epitenon is a fine connective tissue sheath, it is continuous throughout on its inner surface with the endotenon and surrounds the whole tendon.

microfibrils, fibrils, and fibers. A group of fibers constitutes a fascicle. The fascicles unite to form bundles, and are surrounded by the endotenon. The endotenon is a mesh of elastin-rich, loose connective tissue that holds the bundles together and allows some movement of the bundles relative to each other. It carries blood vessels, lymphatics, and nerves. Fascicles are the smallest collagenous structure that can be tested biomechanically [38]. The fascicles can be demonstrated by ultrasound and MRI [39]. A fine connective tissue sheath, the epitenon, is continuous throughout on its inner surface with the endotenon and surrounds the whole tendon (Fig. 11).

Blood supply

The blood supply of tendons is variable, and usually is divided into three regions: the musculo-tendinous junction, the length of the tendon, and the tendon–bone junction. Blood vessels originate from vessels in the perimysium, periosteum, and by way of the paratenon and mesotenon. The Achilles tendon is supplied at its musculotendinous junction, along the length of the tendon, and at its junction with bone. The blood supply consists mainly of longitudinal arteries that course the length of the tendon. The area of lowest vascularity in the Achilles tendon is 2 cm to 6 cm above the insertion of the tendon (Fig. 12) [40,41,43,45–47].

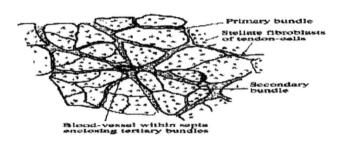

Fig. 12. The area of lowest vascularity in the Achilles tendon is 2 cm to 6 cm above the insertion of the tendon.

The blood supply to the musculo-tendinous junction is from the superficial vessels in the surrounding tissues. Small arteries branch and supply muscles and tendons, but there is no anastomosis between the capillaries.

The main blood supply to the middle portion of the tendon is by way of the paratenon The small blood vessels in the paratenon run transversely toward the tendon and branch several times before running parallel to the long axis of the tendon. The vessels enter the tendon along the endotenon; the arterioles run longitudinally flanked by two venules. Capillaries loop from the arterioles to the venules, but they do not penetrate the collagen bundles. The blood supply of the Achilles tendon mainly arises from the paratenon anterior to the tendon from where vessels run into the tendon [41]. A recurrent branch of the posterior tibial artery supplies the proximal part of the tendon, whereas the distal part is vascularized by the rete arteriosum calcaneare, and supplied by the fibular and posterior tibial arteries. An avascular area can be seen close to the insertion of the tendon to the calcaneus. Three regions with different vascular density are present in the Achilles tendon. The distal part of the Achilles tendon had a vascular density of 56.6 vessels/cm^2. In the middle portion of the tendon, the vascular density was 28.2 vessels/cm^2 [21,29]. The proximal part of the tendon had a vascular density of 73.4 vessels/cm^2.

Vessels that supply the bone–tendon junction supply the lower third of the tendon. There are no direct communications between the vessels because of the fibro-cartilaginous layer between the tendon and bone, but there is some indirect anastomosis between the vessels. The Achilles tendon often is injured through rupture and overuse [10,16,40,42,44,45,47]. The pathogenesis of rupture might involve the pattern of its blood supply. Ahmed et al [45] investigated the blood supply in 12 human cadaveric specimens. Qualitative and quantitative histologic analyses showed that the Achilles tendon has a poor blood supply throughout its length, as determined by the small number of blood vessels per cross-sectional area. This may have been due to the age of the cadavers. The blood supply to tendons also decreases with age. In light of these findings, it is suggested that poor vascularity may prevent adequate tissue repair following trauma, and lead to further weakening of the tendon. The blood flow in the peri-tendinous space increased—during dynamic calf muscle exercise—four-fold from rest to exercise 5 cm from the insertion, but only two-fold at 2 cm from the insertion [44].

Nerve supply

Tendons are supplied by sensory nerves from the overlying superficial nerves or from nearby deep nerves, the tibial nerve, and its branches [23]. The nerve supply is largely, if not exclusively, afferent [48], The afferent receptors are found near the musculo-tendinous junction [23], either on the surface or in the tendon. The nerves tend to form a longitudinal plexus and enter by way of the septa of the endotenon or the mesotenon if there is a synovial sheath.

Branches also pass from the paratenon by way of the epitenon to reach the surface or the interior of a tendon [14,49].

There are four types of receptors. Type I, Ruffini corpuscles are pressure receptors that are sensitive to stretch but adapt slowly [50]. Ruffini corpuscles are oval, 200 μm by 400 μm in diameter. Type II, Vater-Paccinian corpuscles are activated by any movement. Type III, the Golgi tendon organs, are mechano-receptors. They consist of unmyelinated nerve endings that are encapsulated by endoneurial tissue. They lie in series with the extrafusal fibers and monitor increases in muscle tension, rather than length. The Golgi tendon organ is 100 μm in diameter and 500 μm in length. The tendon fiber is less compact here than in the rest of the tendon. Endoneurial tissue encapsulates the unmyelinated nerve fibers. The lamellated corpuscles respond to stimuli that are transmitted by the surrounding tissues (eg, pressure, produced by muscle contraction). The amount of pressure depends on the force of contraction. They may provide a more finely tuned feedback. Type IV receptors are the free nerve endings that act as pain receptors [14].

References

[1] Williams PC, Warwick R, Dyson M, et al, editors. Gray's anatomy. 37th edition. London; 1993.
[2] Warwick R, Williams PC, editors. Gray's anatomy. 35th edition. Edinburgh (Scotland): Longmans; 1973.
[3] Williams SK, Brage M. Heel pain—plantar fasciitis and Achilles enthesopathy. Clin Sports Med 2004;23:123–44.
[4] Soma CA, Mandelbaum BR. Achilles tendon disorders. Clin Sports Med 1994;13:811–23.
[5] Clement DB, Taunton J, Smart GW. A survey of overuse running injuries. Physician Sportsmed 1981;9:47–58.
[6] Smart GW, Taunton JE, Clement DB. Achilles tendon disorders in runners: a review. Med Sci Sports Exerc 1980;12:231–43.
[7] Johansson C. Injuries in elite orienteers. Am J Sports Med 1986;14(5):410–5.
[8] Jones DC. Retrocalcaneal bursitis and insertional tendonitis. Sports Med Arthroscopy Rev 1994;2.
[9] Komi PV. Relevance of in vivo force measurements to human biomechanics. J Biomech 1990;23(Suppl 1):23–4.
[10] Schepsis AA. Achilles tendon disorders in athletes. Am J Sports Med 2002;30(2):287–305.
[11] Maffulli N, Regine R, Angelillo M, et al. Ultrasound diagnosis of Achilles tendon pathology in runners. Br J Sports Med 1987;21(4):158–62.
[12] Maffulli N, Irwin AS, Kenward MG, et al. Achilles tendon rupture and sciatica: a possible correlation. Br J Sports Med 1998;32(2):174–7.
[13] Maffuli N. Rupture of the Achilles tendon. J Bone Joint Surg 1999;81A:1019–36.
[14] Jozsa G, Kannus P. Human tendons Anatomy and Physiology. Human Kinetics 1997.
[15] Kader D, Saxena A, Movin T, et al. Achilles tendinopathy: some aspects of basic science and clinical management. Br J Sports Med 2002;36:239–49.
[16] Kvist M. Achilles tendon overuse injuries [doctoral dissertation]. Turku (Finalnd): University of Turku; 1991.
[17] Kvist M. Achilles tendon injuries in athletes. Sports Med 1994;18:173–201.
[18] Wilder RP, Sethi S. Overuse injuries: tendinopathies, stress fractures, compartment syndrome and shin splints. Clin Sports Med 2004;23:55–81.

[19] Plastanga NP, Field D, Soames R. Anatomy and human movement structure and function. 2nd edition. 1994.

[20] Last RJ. Anatomy, regional and applied. 7th edition. 1984.

[21] Hollinshead WH. Anatomy for surgeons, vol. 3. The back and limbs. 2nd edition. Harper and Row Publishers; 1969.

[22] Kaplan EB. The fabellofibular ligament and the short lateral ligaments of the knee. J Bone Joint Surg 1961;43-A:169–79.

[23] O'Brien M. Functional anatomy and physiology of tendons. Clin Sports Med 1992;11(3): 505–20.

[24] Curwin S, Standish WD. Tendonitis: its etiology and treatment. Lexington (MA): Collamore Press; 1984.

[25] Cummins EJ, Anson BJ, Carr BW, et al. The structure of the calcaneal (Achilles) in relation to orthopaedic surgery. Surg Gynaecol Obst 1946;83:107.

[26] Wood Jones F. Structure and function as seen in the foot. Baillere, Tindall and Cox; 1944.

[27] Barfred T. Experimental rupture of Achilles tendon. Acta Orthop Scand 1971;42:528–43.

[28] Benjamin M, Evans EJ, Copp L. The histology of tendon attachment to bone in man. J Anat 1986;149:89–100.

[29] Leadbetter WB, Mooar PA, Lane GJ, et al. The surgical treatment of tendonitis. Clin Sports Med 1992;11(3):679–712.

[30] Allenmark C. Partial Achilles tendon tears. Clin Sports Med 1992;11(4):759–69.

[31] Snow SW, Bonne WH, Di Carlo E, et al. Anatomy of the Achilles tendon and plantar fascia in relation to the calcaneus in various age groups. Foot Ankle Int 1995;16:418–21.

[32] Williams JGP. Achilles tendon injuries in sport. Sports Med 1986;3:114–35.

[33] Kvist M, Jozsa L, Jarvinen M, et al. Chronic Achilles paratenonitis in athletes: a histologic and histochemical study. Pathology 1987;19:1–11.

[34] Romanelli DA, Almekinders LC, Mandelbaum BR. Achilles rupture in the athlete: current science and treatment. Sports Med Arthroscopy Rev 2000;8:377–86.

[35] Kastelic J, Galeski A, Baer E. The multi composite structure of tendon. Conn Tissue Res 1978;6:11–23.

[36] Jozsa L, Kannus P, Balint JB, et al. Three-dimensional structure of tendons. Acta Anat (Basel) 1991;142:306–12.

[37] Amiel D, Billings E, Akeson WH. Ligament structure, chemistry and physiology. In: Daniel D, editor. Knee ligaments: structure function, injury and repair. New York: Raven Press; 1990. p. 77–91.

[38] Butler DL, Grood ES, Noyes FR, et al. Biomechanics of ligaments and tendons. Exerc Sport Sci Rev 1978;6:125–82.

[39] Read JW, Perduto AJ. Tendon imaging: ultrasound and MRI. Sports Med Arthroscopy Rev 2000;8:32–55.

[40] Lagergen C, Lindholm A. Vascular distribution in Achilles tendon—an angiographic study. Acta Chir Scand 1958;116:491–5.

[41] Zantop T, Tillmann B, Petersen W. Quantitative assessment of blood vessels of the human Achilles tendon: an immunohistochemical cadaver study. Arch Orthop Trauma Surg 2003; 123(9):501–4.

[42] Galloway MT, Jokl P, Dayton OW. Achilles tendon overuse injuries. Clin Sports Med 1992; 11:771–82.

[43] Kvist M, Jozsa L, Jarvinen M. Vascular changes in the ruptured Achilles tendon and paratenon. Int Orthop 1992;16(4):377–82.

[44] Langberg H, Bulow J, Kjaer M. Blood flows in the peritendinous space of the human Achilles tendon during exercise. Acta Physiol Scand 1998;163(2):149–53.

[45] Ahmed IM, Lagopoulos M, McConnell P, et al. Blood supply of the Achilles tendon. J Orthop Res 1998;16(5):591–6.

[46] Carr AJ, Norris SH. The blood supply of the calcaneal tendon. J Bone Joint Surg Br 1989; 71(1):100–1.

[47] Astrom M, Westlin N. Blood flow in the human Achilles tendon assessed by laser Doppler flowmetry. J Orthop Res 1994;12(2):246–52.

[48] Stilwell DL. The innervation of tendons and aponeurosis. Am J Anat 1957;100:289–311.

[49] Ippolito E, Postacchini F. Anatomy. In: Perugia L, Postacchini F, Ippolito E, editors. The tendons: biology-pathology-clinical aspects. Milano (Italy): Editrice Kurtis; 1986. p. 9–36.

[50] Freeman MAR, Wyke B. The innervation of the knee joint. An anatomical and histological study in cats. J Anat 1967;101:505–32.

ELSEVIER
SAUNDERS

Foot Ankle Clin N Am
10 (2005) 239–254

FOOT AND
ANKLE CLINICS

Imaging of the Achilles Tendon

Robert R. Bleakney, MB, BCH, MRAD, FRCR*,
Lawrence M. White, MD, FRCP(C)

*Joint Department of Medical Imaging, University Health Network, and Mount Sinai Hospitals,
5th Floor, University of Toronto, 600 University Avenue, Toronto, Ontario, M5G 1X5, Canada*

The imaging modalities that are used most commonly in the diagnostic evaluation of the Achilles tendon include conventional radiography, ultrasonography, and MRI. Imaging of the Achilles tendon plays a critical role in the diagnostic evaluation and assessment of patients who have clinical symptoms and findings of suspected Achilles origin, in the documentation and differential assessment of disease, and in the staging of the extent and severity of disease present. Imaging also may provide important information regarding the temporal changes of pathologic findings following therapeutic intervention, and, in some instances, may provide prognostic information regarding ultimate tendon function. This article reviews the normal and pathologic imaging features of the Achilles tendon and highlights the potential usefulness and limitations of various imaging techniques in the noninvasive assessment of the tendon and the potential impact of imaging findings on clinical patient care.

Although conventional radiography is the mainstay of bone and joint imaging, particularly in trauma, it lacks soft tissue contrast, and thus, gives limited information regarding soft tissue structures. As a result, cross-sectional imaging, such as ultrasound and MRI, with their excellent soft tissue contrast imaging capabilities, have become the modalities of choice for investigation of the Achilles tendon. In contrast to these cross-sectional imaging modalities, however, conventional radiography is fast, inexpensive, readily available, and may provide important information regarding the Achilles tendon and adjacent structures [1]. On conventional radiography with proper positioning, the Achilles tendon has

---

* Corresponding author. Department of Medical Imaging, 5th Floor, Mount Sinai Hospital, 600 University Avenue, Toronto, Ontario, M5G 1X5, Canada.
E-mail address: rbleakney@mtsinai.on.ca (R.R. Bleakney).

foot.theclinics.com

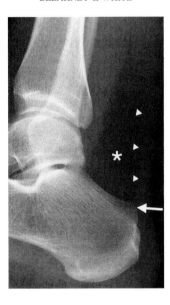

Fig. 1. Lateral conventional radiograph of a normal ankle demonstrating a well-defined anterior margin of the Achilles tendon (*arrowheads*), the pre-Achilles/Kager's fat pad (*), and the retro-calcaneal bursal recess (*solid arrow*).

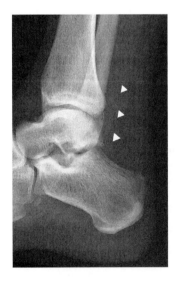

Fig. 2. Lateral conventional radiograph of an ankle following rupture of the Achilles tendon. Note thickening of the Achilles tendon, loss of the normal sharp anterior margin (*arrowheads*) and effacement of the pre-Achilles/Kager's fat pad.

well-defined margins, particularly anteriorly, as a result of the interface between the anterior surface of the tendon and the pre-Achilles fat pad (Kager's triangle) (Fig. 1) [2]. Rupture of the Achilles tendon or Achilles tendinopathy may be associated with edema or hemorrhage which may obscure this sharp interface between the tendon and adjacent fat (Fig. 2) [2].

The normal Achilles tendon should be no more than 8 mm thick, being thickest proximally and tapering in its distal third to its insertion upon the calcaneal tubercle. The normal retrocalcaneal bursal recess should create a radiolucency—anterior to the distal insertional fibers of the Achilles tendon— that extends at least 2 mm below the superior surface of the calcaneus (see Fig. 1) [3]. Bursitis or thickening of the tendon may obliterate this normal radiolucency (Fig. 3). If adjacent erosions are seen to the posterior calcaneus (Fig. 4), then an underlying inflammatory arthritis, such as rheumatoid arthritis or psoriatic arthritis, should be considered [3]. Conventional radiography also is sensitive to the presence of calcification or ossification. Ossification of the Achilles tendon is rare; it is characterized by the presence of an ossific mass that is contained within the substance of the tendon and usually is seen in the clinical setting of previous Achilles tendon rupture or chronic Achilles tendinopathy (Fig. 5) [4].

Musculoskeletal ultrasound (MSK US) is being used more frequently, particularly in Europe. Continual improvement in the technology with the advent of higher frequency transducers (7–15 MHz), smaller footprint probes, power Doppler, extended field of view capabilities [5], three-dimensional imaging, and tissue harmonics [6], is responsible, in part, for this popularity. MSK US has

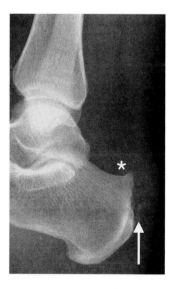

Fig. 3. Lateral conventional radiograph of an ankle showing a thickened distal Achilles tendon, loss of the normal retro-calcaneal bursal recess, dystrophic insertional ossification (*solid arrow*), and a retro-calcaneal bursitis, replacing the normal low attenuation fat pad (*).

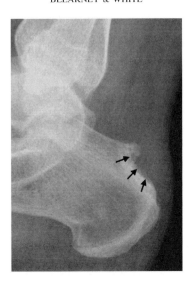

Fig. 4. Lateral conventional radiograph of an ankle in a patient who has psoriatic arthritis illustrating thickening of the distal Achilles tendon and adjacent erosion of the posterior calcaneus (*solid arrows*).

several essential advantages over MRI; it is readily assessable, has a quick scan time, and better patient tolerability. MSK US also allows easy contralateral comparison. Also, the personal interaction with the patient, which can create a more directed examination, is tailored to the investigation of specific clinical complaints or symptoms; however, MSK US is operator dependent, with a long learning curve. Proper training and experience are required for accurate and efficient use of this modality in clinical practice. Higher frequency transducers provide better spatial resolution, and thus, more detailed delineation of normal

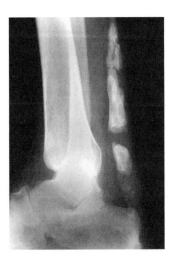

Fig. 5. Lateral conventional radiograph showing ossification of the Achilles tendon.

and abnormal tissues, but are of little use in the assessment of deeper structures because of poor return of echoes. Superficial tendons, and in particular, the Achilles tendon, are ideally suited to evaluation by MSK US. Over the last 20 years, MSK US has been used increasingly in the investigation of the Achilles tendon from the diagnosis of tendinopathy and rupture to posttreatment follow-up [7–18].

Ultrasonographic evaluation of tendons should be performed in longitudinal and transverse planes [9,19]. For optimal imaging, it is necessary to orientate the ultrasound probe so that the ultrasonic waves reach the tendon perpendicularly. The highly ordered pattern of parallel collagen tendon fibers shows the highest echogenicity when examined perpendicular to the ultrasound beam. If this is not the case, most of the reflected ultrasonic waves will not be received by the transducer and tendons will appear hypoechoic or anechoic (Fig. 6). This angle-dependent appearance of tissue structures is referred to as acoustic fiber anisotropy [20]. Artifacts from fiber anisotropy should not be interpreted as pathologic. Awareness of the normal curvature of tendons and proper ultrasono-graphic investigation, including dynamic real-time imaging in more than one plane, are essential to avoid this potential imaging pitfall [21]. Aside from its insertion onto the calcaneus, the Achilles tendon has a straight course compared with other ankle tendons, and thus, is less susceptible to anisotropy at imaging evaluation. Nevertheless, careful examination of the Achilles, particularly at the tendon's calcaneal insertion, with cranial and caudal angulation of the probe is necessary to determine the tendon integrity.

The normal Achilles tendon should have an echogenic pattern of parallel fibrillar lines in the longitudinal plane and an echogenic round-to-ovoid shape in the transverse plane (Fig. 7). The number of echogenic lines that is visible in the tendon with ultrasound is simply a correlate of the ultrasound probe frequency [22]. Two bursae can be present around the area of insertion of the Achilles tendon onto the calcaneus. They can be well-delineated at ultrasonography. The pre-Achilles bursa, also referred to as the retrocalcaneal bursa, lies deep to the

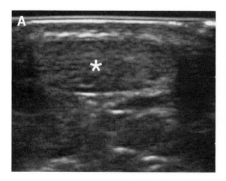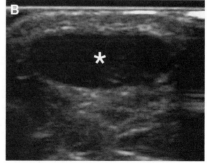

Fig. 6. Transverse ultrasound images of a normal Achilles tendon. (*A*) Probe orientated at 90° to the tendon demonstrating a normal echobright tendon (*). (*B*) Probe angled off perpendicular to the tendon demonstrating a hypoechoic (*dark*) tendon (*).

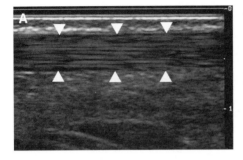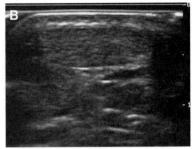

Fig. 7. (*A*) Longitudinal ultrasonographic image of a normal Achilles tendon. Note the echogenic, parallel fibrillar pattern (*between arrowheads*). (*B*) Transverse ultrasonographic image of a normal Achilles tendon showing echogenic ovoid shape.

Achilles tendon between the Achilles tendon and the subjacent calcaneus (Fig. 8). This bursa is seen commonly in normal subjects and varies considerably in appearance and relative dimensions with flexion and extension at the ankle joint [15]. The superficial tendo-Achilles bursa or retro-Achilles bursa is an acquired bursa that occurs in the potential soft tissue interval superficial to the distal tendon, between it and the subcutaneous tissues. This bursa is not seen in normal individuals; typically, its presence is posttraumatic or inflammatory (see Fig. 8) [23]. Proximal to its calcaneal insertion, the Achilles tendon lies immediately superficial to the pre-Achilles fat pad, a triangular area of adipose tissue that also is known as Kager's triangle. On ultrasound imaging, the pre-Achilles fat pad illustrates low mottled echogenicity relative to the normally echogenic tendon. Further anterior to this pre-Achilles fat pad is the deep flexor compartment of the calf—predominantly composed of the flexor hallucis longus muscle—which overlies the echobright bony echoes of the posterior tibia and talus (Fig. 9). On transverse imaging, the normal Achilles tendon has a flat to concave anterior surface and measures 4 mm to 6 mm in anterior to posterior (AP) diameter [8,12,24,25]. Although 6 mm generally is accepted as the upper limit of normal

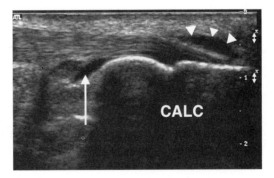

Fig. 8. Longitudinal ultrasonographic image of the Achilles tendon insertion onto the calcaneus (CALC), demonstrating a normal retro-calcaneal bursa (*solid arrow*) and a retro-Achilles bursa (*arrowheads*).

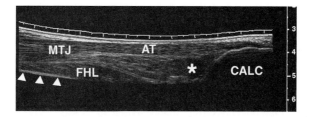

Fig. 9. Longitudinal extended field of view ultrasonographic image of the Achilles tendon (AT), extending from its soleal musculotendinous junction (MTJ) to its insertion onto the calcaneus. Deep to the Achilles is the flexor hallucis longis (FHL), tibial cortex (*arrowheads*), and Kager's fat pad (*).

for AP dimension, the measurement can vary as the result of anatomic variation in the shape of the Achilles tendon [25].

Focal or diffuse thickening of the Achilles tendon is seen most commonly in association with tendinopathy (Fig. 10). The tendon thickness may range from 7 mm to 16 mm in patients who have a clinical diagnosis of tendinopathy [8]. Similarly, in athletes who have the clinical diagnosis of Achilles tendinopathy, the affected tendons were an average of 78% thicker than the contralateral unaffected tendon [14]. Focal hypoechoic areas within the normally echobright tendon are believed to represent areas of tendinopathy [10,26]. Many of the so-called "spontaneous tendon ruptures" are due to progressive degeneration of the tendon [27]. Thickening of the tendon and focal hypoechoic areas are seen

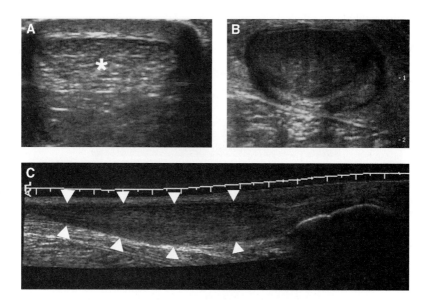

Fig. 10. (*A*) Normal transverse ultrasonographic image of the Achilles tendon (*). (*B*) Transverse ultrasonographic image of an Achilles tendinopathy. The tendon is thickened, heterogeneous, and hypoechoic. (*C*) Longitudinal extended field of view ultrasonographic image of Achilles tendinopathy demonstrating fusiform thickening of the Achilles tendon (*arrowheads*).

with tendinopathy and partial tearing; this makes the differentiation between the two difficult [1,26,28]. Åström et al [26] proposed that thickening of the tendon to greater than 10 mm and severe intratendinous abnormalities indirectly suggest partial rupture; however, true partial tears are rare at surgery, and imaging appearance can be misleading.

Ultrasound is accurate in the diagnosis of full thickness tears of the Achilles tendon [11,28]. Paavola et al [28] correctly diagnosed 25 of 26 full thickness tears before surgery, and Hartgerink et al [11] showed that ultrasound can be effective in the differentiation of full versus partial thickness tears or tendinopathy, with a sensitivity and specificity of 100% and 83%, respectively, and an accuracy of 92%. Undetectable tendon at the site of injury, tendon retraction, and posterior acoustic shadowing at the site of a tendon tear have been described as ultrasonographic signs of a full thickness tear (Fig. 11) [11,12]. Posterior acoustic shadowing deep to the torn tendon margins is believed to occur secondary to sound beam refraction by frayed/torn tendon ends [12]. A potential pitfall in the ultrasound evaluation of a torn Achilles tendon is visualization of an intact plantaris tendon medial to the torn fibers of the Achilles. The normal plantaris tendon may be mistaken for residual intact Achilles tendon fibers, and can lead to a false diagnosis of a high-grade partial tear, rather than a complete tendon tear [11,29]. Dynamic ultrasound assessment of an Achilles tendon rupture can reveal whether the retracted torn tendon ends can be approximated on plantarflexion. This may be of use when deciding between conservative and surgical treatment.

Following successful management of Achilles tendon rupture and tendinopathy, tendon abnormalities can persist on ultrasound although the patient may be asymptomatic. Following Achilles tendon rupture that is treated conservatively or operatively, the tendon can continue to appear thickened and irregular

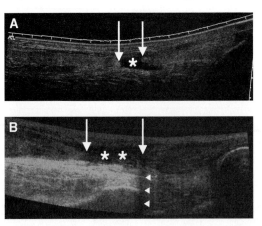

Fig. 11. (A) Longitudinal extended field of view ultrasonographic image of a complete tendon tear showing the gap in the tendon (*) and the torn tendon ends (solid arrows). (B) Longitudinal extended field of view ultrasonographic image of a complete tendon tear. Note more retraction, compared with (A), with a larger gap in the tendon (*), torn tendon ends (solid arrows) and the acoustic shadowing deep to the torn distal tendon end (arrowheads).

with focal hypoechoic areas on ultrasound evaluation [8,16,30–32]. Rupp et al [16] tried to correlate long-term clinical outcome after surgery for Achilles tendon rupture with ultrasound morphology of the tendon. They found that although ultrasound is able to reveal long-lasting changes of the morphology of the tendon, it was of limited value in evaluation of the functional result. Calcifications also may occur at the site of a previous tear; they are seen as hyperechoic areas that cast acoustic shadowing (Fig. 12) [8,30,31]. Despite the ability of ultrasound to depict structural abnormalities of the Achilles tendon accurately, only moderate correlation exists between ultrasound appearance and clinical assessment of chronic Achilles tendinopathy [33]. In addition, the baseline ultrasound appearance of the tendon, in the setting of chronic tendinopathy, was not an accurate predictor of subsequent clinical outcome [33]. Conversely, tendon inhomogeneity can be used to predict clinical outcome in painful Achilles tendons [34,35]. Nehrer et al [36] additionally reported that patients who had a clinical diagnosis of Achilles tendinopathy and a normal ultrasound appearance of the Achilles had a significantly better clinical outcome than individuals who had abnormal findings on ultrasound examination [36]. They also documented that patients who had tendon thickening and focal hypoechoic areas had greater rates of subsequent spontaneous tendon rupture [36].

The recent addition of color and power Doppler imaging to ultrasound has allowed for the noninvasive study of blood flow and vascularity within and surrounding the Achilles tendon. In patellar tendinopathy, color Doppler demonstrated increased vascularity in the abnormal tendon which suggests neovascularization [37]. Zanetti et al [35] demonstrated that the presence of neovascularization usually is a specific sign for a painful tendon; however, the presence of neovascularization did not affect the patient's outcome adversely [35].

The multi-planar imaging capabilities of MRI, combined with its excellent soft tissue contrast characteristics, make it ideally suited for imaging of the Achilles tendon. Sagittal and axial planes are most useful in the evaluation of the Achilles tendon and commonly use a combination of T1- and T2-weighted imaging sequences [38,39]. In general, T1- or intermediate-weighted sequences provide optimal delineation of anatomic detail, whereas T2-weighted sequences are most sensitive to the abnormal increase in water signal that accompanies most patho-

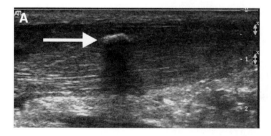 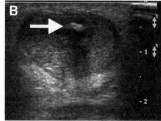

Fig. 12. Longitudinal (*A*) and transverse (*B*) ultrasonographic images of a previously torn Achilles tendon. There is a focal echogenic (*bright*) area of calcification (*arrows*) with posterior acoustic shadowing. The Achilles tendon is thickened, hypoechoic, and heterogeneous.

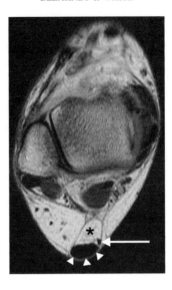

Fig. 13. Axial T2-weighted sequence of a normal ankle, demonstrating a normal Achilles tendon (*arrowheads*), adjacent plantaris tendon (*solid arrow*), and Kager's fat pad (*).

logic conditions of the tendon [40]. Short tau inversion recovery (STIR) and fat saturation T2-weighted sequences also may serve to increase signal contrast between free water and the surrounding fat and adjacent tendon. The normal average AP dimension of the Achilles tendon on MRI is 6 mm [25]; on axial imaging, the anterior aspect of the tendon should be flat to concave (Fig. 13). The length of the Achilles tendon is variable and ranges from 20 mm to 120 mm

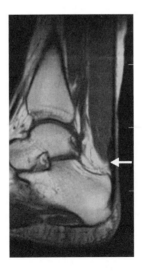

Fig. 14. Sagittal T1-weighted image of the ankle showing an accessory soleus tendon with a distal insertion onto the anterior margin of the Achilles tendon (*solid arrow*).

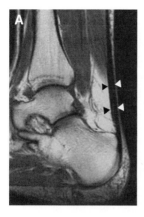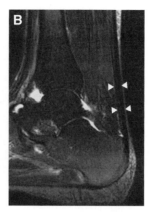

Fig. 15. Sagittal T1- (*A*) and T2-weighted images with fat saturation (*B*) images, of a normal Achilles tendon. Note the parallel anterior and posterior tendon surfaces (*arrowheads*) and its low signal (*black*) appearance on both sequences.

between the musculotendinous origin and the calcaneal insertion of the tendon [41]. The presence of an accessory soleus muscle produces an apparent shorter Achilles tendon, because the accessory soleus may have an insertion directly onto the anterior margin of the Achilles tendon and mimic a more distal musculo-tendinous origin (Fig. 14) [42].

On sagittal magnetic resonance images, the anterior and posterior aspects of the normal Achilles tendon should be parallel distal to the soleus insertion [43]. The normal Achilles tendon is of low signal (black) on all MRI sequences; this reflects its ultrastructural composition of compact parallel arrangements of collagen fibers and its low intrinsic water content (Fig. 15) [25,40,43]. Magic angle phenomenon can cause areas of increased signal within normal tendons that is observed as tendon fibers approach an orientation angle of 55° relative to the main magnetic field, however [44,45]. Although the Achilles tendon has a generally straight course, this effect can occur as the Achilles fibers spiral internally [43]. The magic angle effect usually is seen with echo times of less than 20 millisecond (eg, T1-weighted and proton density/intermediate acquisitions); however, the effect should not be present on T2-weighted (long echo time) acquisitions [45]. Recently, magnetic resonance magic angle imaging was used to image the Achilles tendon. This technique uses the magic angle phenomenon; the Achilles tendon is imaged at 55° relative to the main magnetic field, rather than the normal 0°. In this way, signal becomes detectable within the tendon [46–48]. Using this method, STIR signal change was more apparent, and contrast enhancement was much more evident within the tendon [47].

As with ultrasonographic assessment, a pre-Achilles/retro-calcaneal bursa can be seen in asymptomatic individuals at MRI evaluation; it usually measures no more than 6 mm craniocaudally, 3 mm medial to lateral, and 2 mm anterior to posterior [49]. Achilles paratendinopathy manifests as linear or reticular areas of increased signal on T2-weighted images—paralleling the deep margin

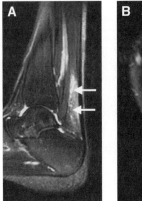
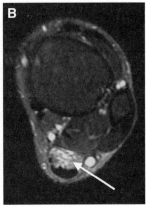

Fig. 16. Sagittal (*A*) and axial (*B*) T2-weighted images with fat saturation showing linear and reticular increase in T2 signal (*solid arrows*) in Kager's fat pad consistent with a peritendinitis.

of the Achilles tendon—that represent areas of edema or increased vascularity (Fig. 16). Ultrasound and MRI evaluation are unreliable in the assessment of the paratenon [26].

At MRI, Achilles tendinopathy is manifest by findings of a fusiform tendon shape, AP tendon thickening, convex bulging of the anterior tendon margin, and areas of increased intratendinous signal on T1- and T2-weighted sequences (Fig. 17) [43,50]. Areas of increased signal within the tendon on T2-weighted sequences are believed to represent more severe areas of collagen disruption [50,51] and partial tearing (Fig. 18) [26]. Marked AP thickening of the tendon to greater than 10 mm also was shown to correlate with pathologic findings of partial tendon tearing [26]. Full-thickness tearing of the Achilles tendon is

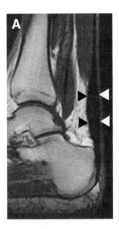
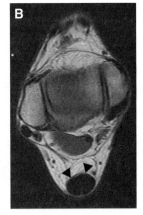

Fig. 17. (*A*) Sagittal T1-weighted image demonstrating fusiform thickening of the Achilles tendon (*arrowheads*). (*B*) Axial T2-weighted image demonstrating a thickened Achilles tendon with a convex anterior border (*arrowheads*).

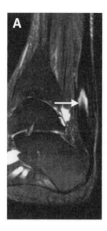
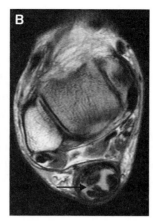

Fig. 18. (*A*) Sagittal T2-weighted image with fat saturation, in a patient who has severe tendinopathy and partial tearing, showing a markedly thickened Achilles tendon with increased T2 signal within the tendon (*solid arrow*). (*B*) Axial T2-weighted image, in the same patient, again demonstrating a thickened AP dimension of the Achilles tendon and areas of increased T2 signal within the tendon (*solid arrow*).

depicted as complete disruption of the tendon fibers with discontinuity of fibers and high-signal intensity within the tendon gap acutely on T2-weighted images (Fig. 19) [52]. As with ultrasound examination, MRI following Achilles tendon repair typically illustrates tendon thickening and intrasubstance imaging heterogeneity [32,51,52]. A decrease in intrasubstance signal and an increased

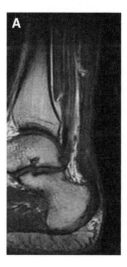
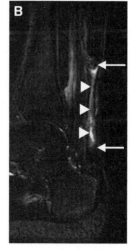

Fig. 19. Sagittal T1 (*A*) and sagittal T2 with fat saturation (*B*) weighted images in a patient who has an Achilles tendon rupture. Note discontinuity of fibers, high signal within the tendon gap (*arrowheads*), and the torn tendon ends (*solid arrows*).

tendon size may progress gradually after surgery over 1 to 2 years; it may reflect the progressive fibrous scar formation at the repair site.

There is some debate as to the usefulness of MRI in examination of the Achilles tendon. Karjalainen et al [50] examined 117 Achilles tendons with MRI and documented the overall sensitivity of MRI in the detection of abnormalities in cases of painful Achilles tendon to be 94%, with a specificity of 81% and overall accuracy of 89%. The interobserver agreement for the MRI findings was good in all categories; however, several investigators demonstrated an overlap in imaging findings in symptomatic and asymptomatic individuals [41,53]. Signal heterogeneity and subtle focal increases in intrasubstance signal with distal longitudinal striations or small punctate foci of increased T1-weighted signal may represent normal fascial anatomy or small vessels [41]. This fascicular signal should be less apparent on STIR/T2-weighted images and the morphology of the tendon should be normal with a concave anterior surface on axial imaging [54]. Haims et al [53] postulated that in asymptomatic subjects, areas of increased T2-weighted signal may represent asymptomatic tendinopathy/mucoid degeneration; however, areas of intense T2-weighted signal and thickened tendons were associated with chronic symptoms and tears. Unlike ultrasound, Khan et al [33] showed that graded MRI correlated with 12-month clinical outcome in patients who had tendinopathy.

Summary

The Achilles tendon is the most commonly injured tendon in the foot and ankle; injuries commonly are related to sports/athletic activities. Imaging modalities that are used most commonly in the diagnostic assessment of the Achilles tendon include conventional radiography, ultrasonography, and MRI. Imaging plays an important role in the documentation and staging of diseases of the Achilles tendon, and provides a noninvasive means of assessing the tendon's response to therapy or progression of disease.

References

[1] Cheung Y, Rosenberg ZS, Magee T, et al. Normal anatomy and pathologic conditions of ankle tendons: current imaging techniques. Radiographics 1992;12:429–44.

[2] Fischer E. Low kilovolt radiography. In: Resnick D, Niwayama G, editors. Diagnosis of bone and joint disorders. Philadelphia: WB Saunders; 1981. p. 367–9.

[3] Resnick D, Feingold DPM, Curd J, et al. Calcaneal abnormalities in articular disorders. Rheumatoid arthritis, ankylosing spondylitis, psoriatic arthritis and Reiter syndrome. Radiology 1977;125:355–66.

[4] Yu JS, Witte D, Resnick D, et al. Ossification of the Achilles tendon: imaging abnormalities in 12 patients. Skeletal Radiol 1994;23(2):127–31.

[5] Barberie JE, Wong AD, Cooperberg PL, et al. Extended field-of-view sonography in musculo-skeletal disorders. AJR Am J Roentgenol 1998;171(3):751–7.

[6] Adler RS. Future and new developments in musculoskeletal ultrasound. Radiol Clin N Am 1999;37:623–31.

[7] Bertolotto M, Perrone R, Martinoli C, et al. High resolution ultrasound anatomy of normal Achilles tendon. Br J Radiol 1995;68(813):986–91.

[8] Fornage BD. Achilles tendon: US examination. Radiology 1986;159(3):759–64.

[9] Fornage BD, Rifkin MD. Ultrasound examination of tendons. Radiol Clin N Am 1988;26(1): 87–107.

[10] Gibbon WW, Cooper JR, Radcliffe GS. Sonographic incidence of tendon microtears in athletes with chronic Achilles tendinosis. Br J Sports Med 1999;33:129–30.

[11] Hartgerink P, Fessell DP, Jacobson JA, et al. Full-versus partial-thickness Achilles tendon tears: sonographic accuracy and characterization in 26 cases with surgical correlation. Radiology 2001;220(2):406–12.

[12] Kainberger FM, Engel A, Barton P, et al. Injury of the Achilles tendon: diagnosis with sonography. AJR Am J Roentgenol 1990;155:1031–6.

[13] Kaplan PA, Matamoros A, Anderson JC. Sonography of the musculoskeletal system. AJR Am J Roentgenol 1990;155:237–45.

[14] Maffulli N, Regine R, Angelillo M, et al. Ultrasound diagnosis of Achilles tendon pathology in runners. Br J Sports Med 1987;21(4):158–62.

[15] Mathieson JR, Connell DG, Cooperberg PL, et al. Sonography of the Achilles tendon and adjacent bursae. AJR Am J Roentgenol 1988;151:127–31.

[16] Rupp S, Tempelhof S, Fritsch E. Ultrasound of the Achilles tendon after surgical repair: morphology and function. Br J Radiol 1995;68:454–8.

[17] O'Reilly MA, Massouh H. Pictorial review: the sonographic diagnosis of pathology in the Achilles tendon. Clin Radiol 1993;48(3):202–6.

[18] Maffulli N, Dymond NP, Capasso G. Ultrasonographic findings in subcutaneous rupture of Achilles tendon. J Sports Med Phys Fitness 1989;29:365–8.

[19] Lin J, Fessell DP, Jacobson JA, et al. An illustrated tutorial of musculoskeletal sonography: part 1, introduction and general principles. AJR Am J Roentgenol 2000;175:637–45.

[20] Dussik KT, Fritch DJ, Kyriazidou M, et al. Measurements of articular tissues with ultrasound. Am J Phys Med 1958;37(3):160–5.

[21] Fornage BD. The hypoechoic normal tendon: a pitfall. J Ultrasound Med 1987;6:19–22.

[22] Martinoli C, Derchi LE, Pastorino C, et al. Analysis of echotexture of tendons with US. Radiology 1993;186(3):839–43.

[23] Frey C, Rosenberg Z, Shereff M, et al. The retrocalcaneal bursa: anatomy and bursography. Foot Ankle 1982;13:203–7.

[24] Civeira F, Castillo JJ, Calvo C, et al. Achilles tendon size by high resolution sonography in healthy population. Med Clin (Barc) 1998;111(2):41–4.

[25] Koivunen-Niemela T, Parkkola K. Anatomy of the Achilles tendon (tendo calcaneus) with respect to tendon thickness measurements. Surg Radiol Anat 1995;17:263–8.

[26] Åström M, Gentz C-F, Nilsson P, et al. Imaging in chronic Achilles tendinopathy: a comparison of ultrasonography, magnetic resonance imaging and surgical findings in 27 histologically verified cases. Skeletal Radiol 1996;25:615–20.

[27] Kainberger F, Mittermaier F, Seidl G, et al. Imaging of tendons—adaptation, degeneration, rupture. Eur J Radiol 1997;25:209–22.

[28] Paavola M, Paakkala T, Kannus P, et al. Ultrasonography in the differential diagnosis of Achilles tendon injuries and related disorders. A comparison between pre-operative ultrasonography and surgical findings. Acta Radiol 1998;39(6):612–9.

[29] Patel RS, Fessell DP, Jacobson JA, et al. Artifacts, anatomic variants, and pitfalls in sonography of the foot and ankle. AJR Am J Roentgenol 2002;178:1247–54.

[30] Hollenberg GM, Adams MJ, Weinberg EP. Sonographic appearance of nonoperatively treated Achilles tendon ruptures. Skeletal Radiol 2000;29:259–64.

[31] Bleakney RR, Tallon C, Wong JK, et al. Long-term ultrasonographic features of the Achilles tendon after rupture. Clin J Sport Med 2002;12(5):273–8.

[32] Moller M, Kalebo P, Tiderbrant G, et al. The ultrasonographic appearance of the ruptured

Achilles tendon during healing: a longitudinal evaluation of surgical and nonsurgical treatment, with comparisons to MRI appearance. Knee Surg Sports Traumatol Arthrosc 2002;10:49–56.

[33] Khan KM, Forster BB, Robinson J, et al. Are ultrasound and magnetic resonance imaging of value in assessment of Achilles tendon disorders? A two year prospective study. Br J Sports Med 2003;37:149–53.

[34] Archambault JM, Wiley JP, Bray RC, et al. Can sonography predict the outcome in patients with achillodynia? J Clin Ultrasound 1998;26(7):335–9.

[35] Zanetti M, Metzdorf A, Kundert H-P, et al. Achilles tendons: clinical relevance of neo-vascularization diagnosed with power doppler US. Radiology 2003;227(2):556–60.

[36] Nehrer S, Breitenseher M, Brodner W, et al. Clinical and sonographic evaluation of the risk of rupture in the Achilles tendon. Arch Orthop Trauma Surg 1997;116(1–2):14–8.

[37] Weinberg EP, Adams MJ, Hollenberg GM. Color Doppler sonography of patellar tendinosis. AJR Am J Roentgenol 1998;171(3):743–4.

[38] Quinn SF, Murray WT, Clark RA, et al. Achilles tendon: MR imaging at 1.5 T. Radiology 1987; 164:767–70.

[39] Bencardino JT, Rosenberg ZS, Serrano LF. MR imaging of tendon abnormalities of the foot and ankle. Magn Reson Imaging Clin N Am 2001;9(3):475–92.

[40] Rosenberg ZS, Beltran J, Bencardino JT. From the RSNA Refresher Courses. Radiological Society of North America. MR imaging of the ankle and foot. Radiographics 2000;20:S153–79.

[41] Soila K, Karjalainen P, Aronen HJ, et al. High-resolution MR imaging of the asymptomatic Achilles tendon: new observations. AJR Am J Roentgenol 1999;173:323–8.

[42] Cheung Y, Rosenberg ZS. MR imaging of the accessory muscles around the ankle. Magn Reson Imaging Clin N Am 2001;9(3):465–73.

[43] Schweitzer ME, Karasick D. MR imaging of disorders of the Achilles tendon. AJR Am J Roentgenol 2000;175:613–25.

[44] Erickson SJ, Cox IH, Hyde JS, et al. Effect of tendon orientation on MR imaging signal intensity: a manifestation of the "magic angle" phenomenon. Radiology 1991;181:389–92.

[45] Erickson SJ, Prost RW, Timins ME. "Magic angle" effect: background physics and clinical relevance. Radiology 1993;188:23–5.

[46] Marshall H, Howarth C, Larkman DJ, et al. Contrast-enhanced magic-angle MR imaging of the Achilles tendon. AJR Am J Roentgenol 2002;179(1):187–92.

[47] Oatridge A, Herlihy A, Thomas RW, et al. Magic angle imaging of the Achilles tendon in patients with chronic tendonopathy. Clin Radiol 2003;58(5):384–8.

[48] Oatridge A, Herlihy AH, Thomas RW, et al. Magnetic resonance: magic angle imaging of the Achilles tendon. Lancet 2001;358(9293):1610–1.

[49] Bottger BA, Schweitzer ME, El-Noueam KI, et al. MR imaging of the normal and abnormal retrocalcaneal bursae. AJR Am J Roentgenol 1988;170:1239–41.

[50] Karjalainen PT, Soila K, Aronen HJ, et al. MR imaging of overuse injuries of the Achilles tendon. AJR Am J Roentgenol 2000;175:251–60.

[51] Karjalainen PT, Aronen HJ, Pihlajamäki HK, et al. Magnetic resonance imaging during healing of surgically repaired Achilles tendon ruptures. Am J Sports Med 1997;25:164–71.

[52] Keene JS, Lash EG, Fisher DR, et al. Magnetic resonance imaging of Achilles tendon ruptures. Am J Sports Med 1989;17:333–7.

[53] Haims AH, Schweitzer ME, Patel RS, et al. MR imaging of the Achilles tendon: overlap of findings in symptomatic and asymptomatic individuals. Skeletal Radiol 2000;29:640–5.

[54] Bencardino JT, Rosenberg ZS. Normal variants and pitfalls in MR imaging of the ankle and foot. Magn Reson Imaging Clin N Am 2001;9(3):447–63.

ELSEVIER
SAUNDERS

Foot Ankle Clin N Am
10 (2005) 255–266

FOOT AND
ANKLE CLINICS

Achilles Tendon Disorders: Etiology and Epidemiology

Tero A.H. Järvinen, MD, PhD[a,b,c,*],
Pekka Kannus, MD, PhD[a,b,d],
Nicola Maffulli, MD, MS, PhD, FRCS(Orth)[e],
Karim M. Khan, MD, PhD[f]

[a]*Department of Orthopaedic Surgery, Tampere University Hospital, Tampere, Finland*
[b]*Medical School and the Institute of Medical Technology, University of Tampere, Tampere, Finland*
[c]*The Burnham Institute, 10901 North Torrey Pines Road, La Jolla, CA 92037, USA*
[d]*Accident and Trauma Research Center and the Tampere Research Center of Sports Medicine,
UKK Institute, Tampere, Finland*
[e]*Department of Trauma and Orthopaedic Surgery, Keele University School of Medicine,
Stoke-on-Trent, U.K.*
[f]*Department of Family Practice & School of Human Kinetics, 2150 Western Parkway,
University of British Columbia, Vancouver, British Columbia, Canada V6T 1V6*

The tendinous portion of the gastrocnemius and soleus muscles merge to form the Achilles tendon, which is the largest and strongest tendon in the human body [1,2]. The Achilles tendon has a high capacity to withstand the tensional forces that are created by the movements of the human body.

The number and the incidence of tendon injuries, in general, have increased substantially during the last few decades [1–5]. It is estimated that tendon injuries account for 30% to 50% of all injuries that are related to sports. The increase in tendon problems has been dominated by problems with the Achilles tendon, which are common among athletes and the general public.

* Corresponding author. The Burnham Institute, 10901 North Torrey Pines Road, La Jolla, CA 92037.
E-mail address: tjarvinen@burnham.org (T.A.H. Järvinen).

1083-7515/05/$ – see front matter © 2005 Elsevier Inc. All rights reserved.
doi:10.1016/j.fcl.2005.01.013

Achilles tendon injuries have been divided into spontaneous ruptures and overuse injuries. Generally, Achilles tendon problems arise from two different origins: (1) some symptoms are caused solely by the excessive loading-induced injury or degeneration of the Achilles tendon (without any predisposing systemic diseases); and (2) sometimes a systemic disease, such as rheumatoid arthritis, manifests with Achilles tendon symptoms [1]. Only a minority (~2%) of all Achilles tendon complaints and injuries are a result of a systemic, predisposing disease; most tendon problems in a population can be traced to sports and exercise-related overuse [1,6].

Chronic injuries: Achilles tendinopathy

Epidemiology of Achilles tendinopathy

Many terms have been used to describe (Achilles) tendon disorders. Because of the highly confusing terminology for (Achilles) tendon disorders, it recently was recommended that the clinical syndrome—characterized by a combination of pain and swelling (diffuse or localized) in and around the Achilles tendon, accompanied by impaired performance—should be called Achilles tendinopathy [7,8]. Based on histopathologic findings, tendinopathy can be divided into peritendinitis and tendinosis (tendon degeneration), and these entities may coexist in the same, painful Achilles tendon; however, the division cannot be made reliably in the clinical setting [3,4,7,8]. Some investigators avoid the term "degeneration" because they believe it often is interpreted as meaning an irreversible pathologic process, whereas tendinosis likely is reversible. We do not attribute anything to the term degeneration other than to mean the findings that are seen on histopathologic samples.

Achilles tendon overuse injuries are associated commonly with strenuous physical activities, such as running and jumping [1,3,4,9]. The occurrence of Achilles tendinopathy is highest among individuals who participate in middle- and long-distance running, orienteering, track and field, tennis, badminton, volleyball, and soccer [5,9–17]. Johansson [12] and Lysholm and Wiklander [13] reported an annual incidence of Achilles disorders to be between 7% and 9% in top-level runners.

In the studies with extensive material, the most common clinical diagnosis of Achilles disorders is tendinopathy (55%–65%), followed by insertional problems (retrocalcaneal bursitis and insertional tendinopathy; 20%–25%) [5,9–11,17]. In a cohort study with an 11-year follow-up, Kujala et al [18] found questionnaire-reported Achilles tendon overuse injury in 79 of 269 male orienteering runners (29%) and 7 of 188 controls (4%); the age-adjusted odds ratio was 10.0 in runners compared with controls.

Kvist [5,10] studied the epidemiology of Achilles tendon disorders in a large group of competitive and recreational athletes who had Achilles tendon problems. In this report of 698 patients, 66% had Achilles tendinopathy and 23% had Achilles tendon insertional problems. In 8% of the patients, the injury was located at the myotendinous junction, and 3% of the patients had a complete tendon rupture. Eighty-nine percent of the patients were men. Running was the main sports activity in patients who presented with an Achilles tendon disorder (53%); persons who were runners represented 27% of all patients who were studied in the sports medicine clinic where the research was performed.

Chronic Achilles tendon disorders are more common in older athletes than in young athletes (teenage and child athletes) [19]. In a report of 470 patients who had Achilles tendinopathy and insertional complaints, only 25% of subjects were young athletes and 10% were younger than 14 years; most of these younger patients were diagnosed with calcaneal apophysitis (Sever's disease) [10]. Patients who had unilateral Achilles tendinopathy seem to have a high risk of sustaining Achilles tendinopathy in the uninvolved leg as well; almost half of the patients who had the Achilles tendinopathy (41%) developed symptoms of this in the contralateral leg during the 8-year follow-up [20].

Etiology of Achilles tendinopathy

Sports injuries can be caused by intrinsic or extrinsic factors, either alone or combination [21]. In acute trauma, extrinsic factors predominate, whereas overuse injuries generally are multi-factorial in origin. In chronic tendon disorders, an interaction between these two types of factors is common [21].

The basic etiology of the Achilles tendinopathy is known to be multi-factorial, because several extrinsic and intrinsic factors were identified that predispose to these problems (Boxes 1 and 2; Fig. 1) [21,22]. In the epidemiologic studies, various malalignment of the lower extremity and biomechanical faults are claimed to play a causative role in two thirds of the athletes who had Achilles tendon disorders. Kvist [5,10] found in his large series on chronic Achilles tendon overuse injuries that some kind of predisposing malalignment of the lower extremity was found in 60% of patients who had an Achilles tendon disorder (see Box 1); however, the mechanisms by which these factors contribute to the pathogenesis of Achilles tendinopathy remain in dispute [23]. The most common, and perhaps the most important, malalignment in the ankle is caused by hyperpronation of the foot. Increased foot pronation was proposed to be associated with Achilles tendinopathy [23]. Kvist [5,10] demonstrated that limited subtalar joint mobility and limited range of motion of the ankle joint were more frequent in athletes who had Achilles tendinopathy than in those who had other complaints. In addition, forefoot varus correlates with Achilles tendinopathy [5,10,24,25]. Recently, Kaufman et al [25] observed that increased hindfoot inversion and decreased ankle dorsiflexion with the knee in extension is associated with Achilles tendinopathy.

In addition to hyperpronation and the other aforementioned malalignments, leg length discrepancy is one of the more controversial potential contributing

Box 1. Predisposing intrinsic factors related to Achilles tendinopathy in sports

General factors

   Gender
   Age
   Overweight
   Constitution: weak or strong
   Blood group
   HLA-types
   Predisposing diseases
   Blood supply
      Ischemia
      Hypoxia
      Hyperthermia

Local (anatomic) factors on the lower limb

   Malalignments
      Foot hyper- or hypopronation
      Forefoot varus or valgus
      Hindfoot varus or valgus
      Pes planus or cavus
   Leg length discrepancy
   Muscle weakness and imbalance
   Decreased flexibility
   Joint laxity

factors [21]. The traditional orthopedic view is that discrepancies of less than 20 mm are not clinically important [23]. In elite athletes, however, a discrepancy of more than 5 mm to 6 mm may be symptomatic and, consequently, for a discrepancy of 10 mm or more, a built-up shoe or shoe insert has been recommended to prevent overuse symptoms. It must be recognized that the true occurrence of these proposed biomechanical alterations, their magnitude and, above all, their clinical importance is not well-known [21].

   The importance of muscle weakness and imbalance, as well as disturbed musculotendinous flexibility, in the development of Achilles tendon disorders also is a matter of debate; however, muscular strength, power, endurance, and flexibility are an important part of physical performance, and thus, can be important in the prevention of certain sports injuries, particularly tendon injuries [21]. If the muscle is weak or fatigued, the energy-absorbing capacity of

---

Box 2. Predisposing extrinsic factors related to Achilles tendinopathy in sports

General factors

Therapeutic agents
    Corticosteroids (local and systemic)
Fluoroquinolone
    Antibiotics
    Weight-lowering drugs
Drugs
    Anabolic steroids
Drugs/narcotics
    Cannabis
    Heroin
    Cocaine

Sports-related factors

Excessive loads on the lower extremities
    Speed of movement
    Type of movement
    Number of repetitions
    Footwear/sportswear
    Training surface
Training errors
    Overdistance
    Fast progression
    High intensity
    Fatigue
    Poor technique
Environmental conditions
    Heat or cold
    Humidity
    Altitude
    Wind
Poor equipment

---

the whole muscle–tendon unit is reduced, and the muscle no longer protects the tendon from strain injury and subsequent inflammation and pain [21]. Recently, good short-term improvements have been reported in chronic Achilles tendinosis with heavy-load eccentric training, a rehabilitation program that is based on increasing the length, tensile strength, and force of the muscle–tendon unit

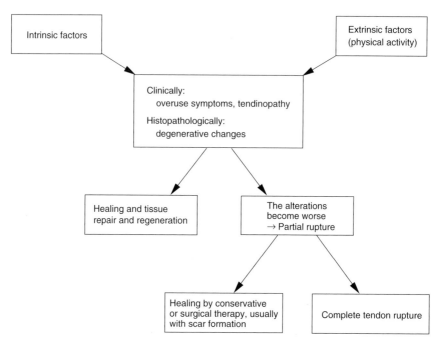

Fig. 1. The pathophysiologic mechanisms of Achilles tendon overuse injuries and disorders, which also may lead to Achilles tendon ruptures.

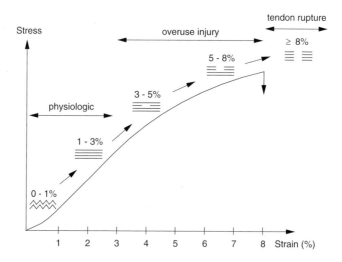

Fig. 2. A schematic presentation of the development of chronic tendon disorders. According to current concepts, repetitive tendon strain (3-5-8% strain) may lead to cumulative fiber microtrauma. If the reparative capacity of the tendon tissue is exceeded, inflammation, edema, pain and tendon degeneration (overuse injury) can ensue.

[26–30]. This concept, however, is open to speculation because the studies do not provide conclusive evidence on whether muscular weakness, imbalance and musculotendinous tightness are the causes or consequences of injuries.

By one definition, an overuse tendon injury is caused by repetitive strain of the affected tendon such that the tendon can no longer endure tensile stress. As a result, tendon fibers begin to disrupt microscopically, and inflammation and pain result (Fig. 2) [21]. Of the extrinsic risk factors, excessive loading of the lower extremities and training errors were said to be present in 60% to 80% of the patients who had Achilles tendon overuse injuries (see Box 2; see Fig. 1) [5,10,22]. The most common of these include running too long a distance, running at too high an intensity, increasing distance too greatly or intensity too rapidly, and performing too much uphill or downhill work [5,10,22,25]. Monotonous, asymmetric, and specialized training, such as running only (ie, without cross-training), as well as poor technique and fatigue are further risk factors for Achilles tendon overuse injuries (see Box 2). Poor environmental conditions, such as cold weather, hard ground surface, and slippery/icy surface also were suggested to promote Achilles tendon problems [1,3,21,23,31]. The lack of high-quality prospective studies limits the strength of the conclusions that can be drawn regarding these extrinsic risk factors.

Achilles tendon ruptures

Epidemiology

Although the incidence of Achilles tendon ruptures is difficult to determine accurately, it is generally agreed that the incidence has increased in the industrialized countries in recent decades [1,2,32–35]. The incidence of ruptures of the Achilles tendon in the city of Oulu, Finland was approximately 18 per 100,000 in 1994 [32], 6 per 100,000 in Scotland in 1994 [33], 37.3 per 100,000 in Denmark (a single county of 220,000 inhabitants) [34], and 17.9 per 100,000 in a single-hospital district (93,000 inhabitants) in eastern Finland [35].

Of all spontaneous tendon ruptures, complete Achilles tendon tears are associated most closely with sports activities. Schönbauer [36] found in his study population that 75% of all Achilles tendon ruptures were related to sports, whereas Plecko and Passl [37] found that the proportion of sports-related Achilles tendon ruptures was 60%. In the material of 430 tendon ruptures that were analyzed by Józsa et al [38], the number of sports-related Achilles ruptures was similar (62%) to the two aforementioned studies, whereas only few (2%) ruptures of other human tendons were sports related.

The distribution of Achilles tendon ruptures according to different sports varies considerably from country to country, according to the national sports traditions. For example, in northern and middle Europe, soccer, tennis, track and field, indoor ball games, downhill skiing, and gymnastics are the most common sports during which the Achilles tendon ruptures take place [1,2]. In North America, American football, basketball, baseball, tennis, and downhill skiing dominate the statistics [1,2].

There also are indications that patients who have spontaneous Achilles tendon ruptures are at increased risk for sustaining a rupture in the contralateral Achilles tendon as well [39].

Etiology of a spontaneous Achilles tendon rupture

The exact cause of Achilles tendon ruptures is not known, because most of the patients who sustain a spontaneous rupture never had any symptoms (tenderness, stiffness, discomfort, diagnosed disease in the region of the ruptured Achilles tendon) before the rupture [1,2,40]. Histopathologic studies on ruptured Achilles tendons show, however, that almost all of these subjects have clear degenerative changes, such as hypoxic and mucoid degeneration, poor vascular supply, tissue and cell necrosis, calcification, and tendolipomatosis, as well as irregular, degenerated collagen fibers at and around the rupture site [41–44]. Furthermore, there is evidence that professional, white-collar workers are overrepresented among patients who have Achilles tendon ruptures [38]. Taking these findings together, it is believed that a sedentary lifestyle (possibly by contributing to poor circulation and subsequent, hypoxic degeneration of the Achilles tendon), together with mechanical factors (sudden or repetitive movements), lead to spontaneous tears of the Achilles tendon [38,40]. A substantial proportion of Achilles tendon ruptures occur in situations in which degeneration of the tendon cannot be traced as an etiologic factor, however. In these cases, the rupture is more a consequence of the remarkably high forces that are involved in the performance (eg, high or triple jump) [1,2].

The biomechanically undesired positions of the ankle and foot, such as forefoot or calcaneal valgus and varus malalignments that cause horizontal, axial, and rotational alterations on the collagen fibers of the Achilles tendon during running are important predisposing factors to rupture [1,2,40].

Generally speaking, patients who have Achilles tendon rupture are younger than those who have other tendon ruptures [6], and there is a clear male predominance among this group of patients [6,38]. Although there are case reports on pre-existing distinct intratendinous diseases as well as a wide range of different generalized concurrent diseases (eg, rheumatoid arthritis, gout, ankylosing spondylitis, chronic uremia, hyperparathyroidism) causing tendon ruptures, they rarely are responsible (<2%) for Achilles tendon rupture and for tendon ruptures, in general [1,6].

Several drugs can cause spontaneous tendon ruptures [40]. Recent literature provides strong evidence that the abuse of anabolic steroids increases the risk of tendon rupture [45]. Since the initial report by Ribard et al [46] that described seven cases of Achilles tendinopathy (three were complicated further by spontaneous rupture of the tendon) after fluoroquinolone antibiotic treatment, several similar cases have been reported around the world [47,48]. Thus, it has become accepted that the fluoroquinolone antibiotics have an unspecific, toxic effect that may cause tendonitis or spontaneous rupture of the Achilles tendon [47].

The issue of corticosteroids and the risk of tendon rupture is controversial in the orthopedic literature [49,50]. In this context, it needs to be emphasized that current literature that was derived from experimental or clinical studies provides no convincing evidence either for or against (intratendinous or peritendinous) corticosteroid injections increasing the risk of tendon rupture (for a review see [50]). Furthermore, rheumatologists have been injecting corticosteroids directly into the tendon tissue for decades without any evidence of increased prevalence of tendon ruptures [51]. A recent study, although small in number of patients treated, indicates that the corticosteroids can be beneficial and safe, even when injected directly into the tendon in athletes who have Achilles tendinopathy [52]. Thus, based on the current evidence on the topic, one plausible explanation for the tendon ruptures that are seen after corticosteroid injection is that rapid pain relief, and consequently, a quick return to strenuous physical activity provides an opportunity for the degenerated tendon to rupture, which merely is a final manifestation of the disease for which the corticosteroids were applied [50].

The role of genetic background of the patient in Achilles tendon rupture is almost unknown. There is evidence of a relationship between ABO blood groups and spontaneous tendon ruptures. A strong association between blood group O and Achilles tendon rupture was identified in a large series of patients in Hungarian and Finnish populations [53,54]. The exact reason for the identified relationship is unknown; the above described relationship has not been found in other populations [55].

Summary

The Achilles tendon is the strongest tendon in the human body. The number and incidence of Achilles tendon overuse injuries and complete, spontaneous ruptures have increased in the industrialized countries during the last decades because of the increased participation in sports.

The most common clinical diagnosis of Achilles overuse injuries is tendinopathy, which is characterized by a combination of pain and swelling in the Achilles tendon accompanied by impaired ability to perform strenuous activities. Achilles tendinopathy is common in sports that require strenuous physical activity. Extrinsic and intrinsic factors contribute to Achilles tendinopathy.

Among the different ruptures of the human tendons, a complete rupture of the Achilles tendon is the one that is associated most closely with sports. Although histopathologic studies showed that ruptured Achilles tendons have clear degenerative changes before the rupture, many Achilles tendon ruptures take place suddenly without any preceding signs or symptoms. Considering that professional white-collar workers are overrepresented among the patients who have Achilles tendon rupture, in conjunction with the degenerative changes that are identified in ruptured tendons, a potential mechanism for the causative effect of a sedentary lifestyle on the increased incidence of spontaneous tendon ruptures has been introduced.

Acknowledgments

This work was supported by grants from the Sigrid Juselius Foundation, Helsinki, Finland; Tampere University Hospital Research Fund; the Research Council for Physical Education and Sport Ministry of Education, Finland; and the AO Foundation, Switzerland.

References

[1] Jozsa L, Kannus P. Human tendons: anatomy, physiology, and pathology. Champaign (IL): Human Kinetics; 1997.

[2] Maffulli N. Rupture of the Achilles tendon. J Bone Joint Surg 1999;81-A(7):1019–36.

[3] Paavola M, Kannus P, Järvinen TAH, et al. Achilles tendinopathy. J Bone Joint Surg 2002; 84-A(11):2062–76.

[4] Maffulli N, Kader D. Tendinopathy of tendo Achillis. J Bone Joint Surg 2002;84-B(1):1–8.

[5] Kvist M. Achilles tendon injuries in athletes. Sports Med 1994;18:173–201.

[6] Kannus P, Jozsa L. Histopathological changes preceding spontaneous rupture of a tendon. A controlled study of 891 patients. J Bone Joint Surg 1991;73-A:1507–25.

[7] Maffulli N, Khan KM, Puddu G. Overuse tendon conditions: time to change a confusing terminology. Arthroscopy 1998;14:840–3.

[8] Khan KM, Cook JL, Kannus P, et al. Time to abandon the "tendinitis" myth. BMJ 2002; 324:626–7.

[9] Järvinen M. Epidemiology of tendon injuries in sports. Clin Sports Med 1992;11(3):493–504.

[10] Kvist M. Achilles tendon injuries in athletes. Ann Chir Gynaecol 1991;80:188–201.

[11] Leppilahti J, Orava S, Karpakka J, et al. Overuse injuries of the Achilles tendon. Ann Chir Gynaecol 1991;80:202–7.

[12] Johansson C. Injuries in elite orienteers. Am J Sports Med 1986;14:410–5.

[13] Lysholm J, Wiklander J. Injuries in runners. Am J Sports Med 1987;15:168–71.

[14] Fahlström M, Lorentzon R, Alfredson H. Painful conditions in the Achilles tendon region in elite badminton players. Am J Sports Med 2002;30:51–4.

[15] Fahlström M, Lorentzon R, Alfredson H. Painful conditions in the Achilles tendon region: a common problem in middle-aged competitive badminton players. Knee Surg Sports Traumatol Arthrosc 2002;10:57–60.

[16] Leppilahti J, Karpakka J, Gorra A, et al. Surgical treatment of overuse injuries to the Achilles tendon. Clin J Sport Med 1994;4:100–7.

[17] Järvinen M. Lower leg overuse injuries in athletes. Knee Surg Sports Traumatol Arthrosc 1993;1(2):126–30.

[18] Kujala UM, Sarna S, Kaprio J, et al. Heart attacks and lower-limb function in master endurance athletes. Med Sci Sports Exerc 1999;31:1041–6.

[19] Kannus P, Niittymäki S, Järvinen M, et al. Sports injuries in elderly athlete: a three-year prospective, controlled study. Age Ageing 1989;18:263–70.

[20] Paavola M, Kannus P, Paakkala T, et al. Long-term prognosis of patients with Achilles tendinopathy. An observational 8-year follow-up study. Am J Sports Med 2000;28:634–42.

[21] Kannus P. Etiology and pathophysiology of chronic tendon disorders in sports. Scand J Sports Med 1997;7(2):78–85.

[22] Järvinen TAH, Kannus P, Józsa L, et al. Achilles tendon injuries. Curr Opin Rheumatol 2001;13(2):150–5.

[23] Nigg BM. The role of impact forces and foot pronation: a new paradigm. Clin J Sports Med 2001;11:2–9.

[24] McCrory JL, Martin DF, Lowery RB, et al. Etiologic factors associated with Achilles tendinitis in runners. Med Sci Sports Exerc 1999;31:1374–81.

[25] Kaufman KR, Brodine SK, Shaffer RA, et al. The effect of foot structure and range of motion on musculoskeletal overuse injuries. Am J Sports Med 1999;27:585–93.

[26] Alfredson H, Pietilä T, Jonsson P, et al. Heavy-load eccentric calf muscle training for the treatment of chronic Achilles tendinosis. Am J Sports Med 1998;26:360–6.

[27] Fahlström M, Jonsson P, Lorentzon R, et al. Chronic Achilles tendon pain treated with eccentric calf-muscle training. Knee Surg Sports Traumatol Arthrosc 2003;11(5):327–33.

[28] Öhberg L, Lorentzon R, Alfredson H. Eccentric training in patients with chronic Achilles tendinosis: normalised tendon structure and decreased thickness at follow up. Br J Sports Med 2004;38(1):8–11.

[29] Shalabi A, Kristoffersen-Wilberg M, Svensson L, et al. Eccentric training of the gastrocnemius-soleus complex in chronic Achilles tendinopathy results in decreased tendon volume and intratendinous signal as evaluated by MRI. Am J Sports Med 2004;32(5):1286–96.

[30] Roos EM, Engström M, Lagerquist A, et al. Clinical improvement after 6 weeks of eccentric exercise in patients with mid-portion Achilles tendinopathy—a randomized trial with 1-year follow-up. Scand J Med Sci Sports 2004;14(5):286–95.

[31] Milgrom C, Finestone A, Zin D, et al. Cold weather training: a risk factor for Achilles paratendinitis among recruits. Foot Ankle Int 2003;24(5):398–401.

[32] Leppilahti J, Puranen J, Orava S. Incidence of Achilles tendon rupture. Acta Orthop Scand 1996;67(3):277–9.

[33] Maffulli N, Waterston SW, Squair J, et al. Changing incidence of Achilles tendon rupture in Scotland: a 15-year study. Clin J Sport Med 1999;9(3):157–60.

[34] Houshian S, Tscherning T, Riegels-Nielsen P. The epidemiology of Achilles tendon rupture in a Danish county. Injury 1998;29(9):651–4.

[35] Nyyssönen T, Luthje P. Achilles tendon ruptures in South-East Finland between 1986–1996, with special reference to epidemiology, complications of surgery and hospital costs. Ann Chir Gynaecol 2000;89(1):53–7.

[36] Schönbauer HR. Diseases of the Achilles tendon. Wien Klin Wschr 1986;98(Suppl 168):1–47.

[37] Plecko M, Passl R. Ruptures of the Achilles tendon: causes and treatment. J Finn Orthop Traumatol 1991;14:201–4.

[38] Józsa L, Kvist M, Balint BJ, et al. The role of recreational sport activity in Achilles tendon rupture. A clinical, pathoanatomical, and sociological study of 292 cases. Am J Sports Med 1989;17(3):338–43.

[39] Aroen A, Helgo D, Granlund OG, et al. Contralateral tendon rupture risk is increased in individuals with a previous Achilles tendon rupture. Scand J Med Sci Sports 2004;14(1):30–3.

[40] Kannus P, Natri A. Aetiology and pathophysiology of tendon ruptures in sports. Scand J Med Sci Sports 1997;7(2):107–12.

[41] Kvist M, Jozsa L, Järvinen M. Vascular changes in the ruptured Achilles tendon and paratenon. Int Orthop 1992;16(4):377–82.

[42] Järvinen TAH, Järvinen TLN, Józsa L, et al. Collagen fibers of the ruptured human tendons display decreased thickness and crimp angle. J Orthop Res 2004;22:1303–9.

[43] Tallon C, Maffulli N, Ewen SW. Ruptured Achilles tendons are significantly more degenerated than tendinopathic tendons. Med Sci Sports Exerc 2001;33(12):1983–90.

[44] Maffulli N, Waterston SW, Ewen SW. Ruptured Achilles tendons show increased lectin stainability. Med Sci Sports Exerc 2002;34(7):1057–64.

[45] Laseter JT, Russell JA. Anabolic steroid-induced tendon pathology: a review of the literature. Med Sci Sports Exerc 1991;23:1–3.

[46] Ribard P, Audisio F, Kahn MF, et al. Seven Achilles tendinitis including 3 complicated by rupture during fluoroquinolone therapy. J Rheumatol 1992;19(9):1479–81.

[47] Khaliq Y, Zhanel GG. Fluoroquinolone-associated tendinopathy: a critical review of the literature. Clin Infect Dis 2003;36(11):1404–10.

[48] Kowatari K, Nakashima K, Ono A, et al. Levofloxacin-induced bilateral Achilles tendon rupture: a case report and review of the literature. J Orthop Sci 2004;9(2):186–90.

[49] Speed CA. Fortnightly review: corticosteroid injections in tendon lesions. BMJ 2001; 323(7309):382–6.

[50] Paavola M, Kannus P, Järvinen TAH, et al. Tendon healing: adverse role of steroid injection—myth or reality. Foot Ankle Clin 2002;7(3):501–13.

[51] Kannus P, Järvinen TLN, Järvinen TAH, et al. Painful Achilles tendon and its treatment [editorial]. Scand J Med Sci Sports 2004;14(2):69–71.

[52] König MJ, Torp-Pedersen S, Qvistgaard E, et al. Preliminary results of colour Doppler guided intratendinous glucocorticoid injection for Achilles tendonitis in 5 patients. Scand J Med Sci Sports 2004;14(2):100–6.

[53] Józsa L, Balint JB, Kannus P, et al. Distribution of blood groups in patients with tendon rupture. An analysis of 832 cases. J Bone Joint Surg Br 1989;71(2):272–4.

[54] Kujala UM, Järvinen M, Natri A, et al. ABO blood groups and musculoskeletal injuries. Injury 1992;23(2):131–3.

[55] Maffulli N, Reaper JA, Waterston SW, et al. ABO blood groups and Achilles tendon rupture in the Grampian region of Scotland. Clin J Sport Med 2000;10(4):269–71.

ELSEVIER
SAUNDERS

Foot Ankle Clin N Am
10 (2005) 267–277

FOOT AND
ANKLE CLINICS

Molecular Events in Tendinopathy: A Role for Metalloproteases

Merzesh Magra, MRCS,
Nicola Maffulli, MD, MS, PhD, FRCS(Orth)*

*Department of Trauma and Orthopaedic Surgery, Keele University School of Medicine,
Thornburrow Drive, Hartshill, Stoke-on-Trent, ST4 7QB Staffordshire, UK*

Matrix metalloproteases (MMPs) may play a major role, possibly combined with factors, such as exercise, nutrition, inflammatory mediators, and reactive oxygen and nitrogen species [1], in tendinopathies.

Tendon structure

The smallest unit of tendon is the fibril, which is primarily made up of collagen [2]. The fibrils aggregate together to form fibers; several fibers make up a fascicle [2]. Fascicles are aligned predominantly with the long axis of the tendon, and are responsible for the tensile strength of the tendon. A small proportion of fibers runs transversely, and in spiral and plait-like formations [3,4]. This complex ultrastructure provides resistance against transverse, shear, and rotational forces that act on the tendon. The fascicles are arranged into bundles, and each bundle is surrounded by a thin layer of loose connective tissue, the endotenon [2]. The bundles are surrounded by a final outer covering, the epitenon [2]. The endotenon and epitenon carry blood vessels, lymphatics, and nerves [2,5]. In the fascicle, the cellular elements are laid out in the extracellular matrix (ECM), which is composed of glycosaminoglycans, proteoglycans, glycoproteins, other noncollagenous proteins and water [6,7]. Tenocytes lie in the ECM. A normal tendon is able to bear a load of 50 N/m^2 to 100 N/m^2 [8], and

* Corresponding author.
E-mail address: n.maffulli@keele.ac.uk (N. Maffulli).

1083-7515/05/$ – see front matter © 2005 Elsevier Inc. All rights reserved.
doi:10.1016/j.fcl.2005.01.012

can be stretched to approximately 4% of its total length before microscopic evidence of rupture of some collagen fibers [9]. Strain in excess of 8% to 12% results in complete tendon rupture [10].

Tendinopathy

Tendinopathy is a broad term that is used to describe disorders in and around tendons. Tendinitis, tendinosis, and paratenonitis all examples of tendinopathy. The pathogenesis of tendinopathy is difficult to study because tendon biopsies rarely are obtained before a tendon is operated on for a chronic tendinopathy or for repair of a rupture. Tendinopathy can be associated with a variety of intrinsic and extrinsic factors (Box 1) [10]. Histopathologic studies on chronic tendinopathy have shown major disorganization and loosening of collagen fibrils [11–13]. Disorganized, haphazard, ineffective healing is a constant feature of chronic tendinopathy. These intratendinous changes may be part of normal ageing [7,13–15]; however, the exact pathophysiologic mechanism is unclear. Heavy physical loading, injury, vibration, infection, smoking, and possibly genetic factors can produce such a histologic picture. Tendinopathy and tendon rupture also can be induced by fluoroquinolone antibiotics [16–18].

Matrix metalloproteases and tissue inhibitors of metalloproteases

Degradation of collagen and other ECM compounds is initiated by MMPs [15]. These are zinc- and calcium-dependent endopeptidases that are secreted from cells in proenzyme form [19]. MMPs are the major enzymes that are involved in remodelling of ECM because of their efficacy at neutral pH and their broad proteolytic capability against the ECM [20].

The MMP family contains 23 members that have some characteristics in common (Table 1) [20]. MMPs are subdivided into four main classes: collagenases, gelatinases, stromelysins, and membrane-type MMPs (MT-MMPs) [21]. MMPs are involved in many physiologic remodelling processes, including wound healing, menstruation, uterine involution, bone growth and development, and angiogenesis [22–24]. Also, MMPs play a role in pathologic processes, such as tumor invasion and metastasis [25–29], multiple sclerosis [30], periodontal disease [31,32], hypertension [33], and arthritis [34–41].

The activity of MMPs is inhibited by tissue inhibitors of metalloproteases (TIMPs) [42,43]. The balance between the activities of MMPs and TIMPs regulates tendon remodelling. An imbalance in MMPs and TIMPs is associated with collagen disturbances in tendons [44]. Cytokines, such as interleukin (IL)-1 and tumor necrosis factor (TNF)-α enhance the production of MMPs [45–47], whereas transforming growth factor (TGF)-β and IL-6 enhance the production of TIMP-1 [48,49].

Box 1. Factors implicated in chronic tendinopathy

Intrinsic factors

    Age
    Vascular perfusion
    Nutrition
    Anatomic variants
        Leg length discrepancy
        Malalignments (eg, genu valgum)
        Bony impingement (eg, acromion)
    Joint laxity
    Muscle weakness/imbalance
    Gender (?)
    Body weight
    Systemic disease

Extrinsic factors

    Occupation
    Sports
    Physical load
        Excessive force
        Repetitive loading
        Abnormal/unusual movement
    Training errors
        Poor technique
        Fast progression
        High intensity
        Fatigue
    Shoes and equipment
    Environmental conditions
        Temperature
        Running surface

Data from Riley G. The pathogenesis of tendinopathy. A molecular perspective. Rheumatology (Oxford) 2004;43:132.

Roles of matrix metalloproteases and tissue inhibitors of metalloproteases in tendinopathy

MMP proenzymes have to be activated before degradation of ECM components [19,50–53]. The mechanism of activation is poorly understood in vivo,

Table 1
The main components of the Matrix Metalloprotease (MMP) Family

Name	Synonym	Degrades
MMP-1	Collagenase-1, interstitial collagenase, fibroblast collagenase	Collagens type III (preferentially), I, and II Type VII, VIII, X
MMP-2	72-kd Gelatinase A 72-kd type IV gelatinase	Gelatin, collagens type IV, V, VII, X, XI Fibronectin, elastin, proteoglycans Synergistic with MMP-1
MMP-3	Stromelysin-1 Transin, proteoglycanase, procollagen-activating factor	Broad substrate specificity Proteoglycans, laminin, fibronectin, gelatin Collagens III, IV, V, IX Core protein of cartilage proteoglycans Activates pro-MMPs
MMP-7	Matrilysin, Pump-1, Small uterine proteinase	Gelatin, proteoglycans, fibronectin, elastin, casein Activates pro-MMP-1
MMP-8	Neutrophil collagenase	Collagens type-1 (preferentially), II, III Aggrecan
MMP-9	92-kd Gelatinase-B, 92-kd Type IV gelatinase	Collagens type IV, V, X, XI Gelatin
MMP-10	Stromelysin-2, transin-2	Gelatin, fibronectin, collagens type III, IV, V Activates pro-MMPs
MMP-11	Stromelysin-3	
MMP-12	Macrophage metalloelastase	
MMP-13	Collagenase-3	Collagens type II (preferentially), I, III Gelatin

Adapted from Goupille P, Jayson MIV, Valat J, et al. Matrix metalloproteinases: the clue to intervertebral disc degeneration? Spine 1998;23(14):1613.

but is likely to involve other enzymes, such as plasmin and MT-MMPs. MMPs with collagenase activity include MMP-1, MMP-2, MMP-8, MMP-13, and MMP-14 [51,54]. Although collagenases play an important role in rheumatologic disorders [55,56], the role of collagenolytic enzymes in degenerative tendinopathy has not been investigated. It is unknown whether MMPs are involved in the turnover of type I collagen in human tendon tissue with mechanical loading.

In animal models, expression of MMP-2 at the edges of an acute tear in the supraspinatus tendon is strongest at 2 weeks, and gradually reduces at 3 and 6 weeks [57]. Hence, it seems that MMP-2 degrades ECM at the tendon edges, and reparative tissue. TIMP-1 is not present in normal tendons, but is expressed in tendon edges at 1 and 2 weeks following acute tears of the supraspinatus tendon; it is expressed in reparative tissue at 2 and 3 weeks. Six weeks after an acute tear, TIMP-1 is not expressed. The expression of TIMP-1 may inhibit excessive degradation of ECM by MMP-2.

In patellar tendinopathy, there is a higher percentage of procollagen type I as compared with normal tendon samples; this reflects a greater collagen turnover in tendinopathy [58]. This suggests that the healing process has started in tendinopathy, but it may not have been able to affect collagenolysis, and this results in disorganized collagen matrix [58]. MMP-1 and TIMP-1 expression in normal tendon is confined to a few cells in the loose connective tissue that surrounds collagen fiber bundles, especially around blood vessels [59]. There is a greater expression of MMP-1 (interstitial collagenase) and suppressed expression of TIMP-1 in tendinopathy [58,59]. In tendinopathic tendons, MMP-1 is expressed in a greater number of tenocytes around blood vessels [59]. In complete tears of rotator cuff tendons, however, there is no significant increase in MMP-1 mRNA expression [60], although the actual activity of MMP-1 may be increased [15]. Conversely, levels of TIMP-1 are greater in normal tendon as compared with tendinopathic tendon [58,59]. This lack of TIMP-1 activity in tendinopathic tendon shifts the delicate balance in favor of greater collagenase activity. This suggests that tendinopathy may be a disorder in the healing of tendon with abnormal cellular responses to injury or repetitive stress which leads to tendon dysfunction, and may result in rupture. Although Choi et al [57] showed an increased expression of TIMP-1 2 weeks following an acute tear, that study was performed on an animal model, and it focused on the relationship between MMP-2 and TIMP-1. It might be possible that TIMP-1 is down-regulated in chronic tendinopathy and up-regulated in acute tears.

There is a down-regulation of MMP-3 in tendinopathic tendons [61,62]. MMP-3 (stromelysin 1) is an MMP with a wide range of substrates, including ECM components, and is a potent activator of other MMPs. Thus, it has the potential to play a major role in the regulation of tendon ECM degradation and tissue remodelling [61]. Although MMP-1 and MMP-3 share homologous gene sequences and similar promoter elements, they do show a differential expression in response to several stimuli, probably by recruiting different sets of transcription factors [63]. Thus, decreased expression of MMP-3, TIMP-1, TIMP-2, TIMP-3, and TIMP-4 is associated with the changes that are seen in tendinopathy [61]. Also, the expression of MMP-3, TIMP-2, TIMP-3, and TIMP-4 mRNA is decreased in torn rotator cuff tendons [60]. Therefore, MMP-3 may play a role in the normal maintenance and remodelling of the rotator cuff tendon; a decrease in normal MMP-3 activity may represent a failure of normal matrix remodelling and maintenance [15]. Also, ruptured supraspinatus tendons show up-regulation of MMP-1 activity with down-regulation of MMP-2 and MMP-3 [15]. Although these findings are potentially significant, causation has not been demonstrated; the mRNA changes that are identified may be secondary to the effects of rotator cuff tearing itself, and not involved in its pathogenesis [60]. The increased expression of MMP-3 may be necessary for correct tissue remodelling and the prevention of tendinopathic changes. The timing of MMP-3 production is also probably critical in this process [61].

In an animal model, Archambault et al [64] showed that tenocytes can alter gene expression in response to fluid flow; up-regulation of the genes for MMP-1 and MMP-3 occurred in response to fluid flow. Thus, shear stress on tenocytes may contribute to tendinopathy by way of the action of MMPs and cyclo-oxygenase II [64]; however, Lavagnino et al [65] showed that stress deprivation up-regulated MMP-1 expression in tenocytes in an animal model. Increasing the cyclic strain frequency eliminated MMP-1 mRNA expression at low-amplitude strain levels [65]. Also, when a static, tensile load is applied to rat tail tendon cells, MMP-1 mRNA expression is inhibited in a dose-dependant manner [66]. Thus, the type of force may influence the expression of MMP-1; shear forces up-regulate MMP-1 [64], whereas cyclical strain and static tensile loads down-regulate MMP-1 [65,66].

The role of tenocytes in the production of MMP-3 has not been investigated, although they synthesize type I and type III collagen. The latter is synthesized in increased amounts after in vitro "wounding" of cultured tenocytes from tendinopathic tendons, but not normal tendons [67]. In tendinopathic tendons, there is a greater proportion of type III collagen as compared with type I collagen. This produces a tissue with reduced tensile strength and increased susceptibility to rupture [67,68].

Certain individuals may be more susceptible to tendon disorders. The production of MMP-3 may be altered in tenocytes that are derived from such individuals; expression of this enzyme may be influenced by polymorphism in the promoter region of the MMP-3 gene. It also is possible that synthesis of natural inhibitors of MMPs, such as TIMP-1, is altered in the tenocytes of these individuals which leads to an imbalance in degradative and reparative changes in tendinopathy.

The supraspinatus tendon is affected frequently by tendinopathy, and most macroscopically normal supraspinatus tendons show microscopic evidence of tendinopathy [69,70]. In ruptured supraspinatus tendons, there is an increased amount of denatured collagen and MMP-1 [15]. An increase in MMP-1 activity and degradation of the collagen fibril network is a potential cause of weakening of the ECM [15]. Lo et al [60] recently showed up-regulation of MMP-13 at the mRNA and protein levels in patients who had complete tears of rotator cuff tendons. Because the rotator cuff is composed primarily of type I collagen [71,72] and MMP-13 is known to degrade type I collagen as efficiently as MMP-1 or MMP-8 [73], MMP-13 may play a role in the tearing of the rotator cuff or its remodelling.

Human flexor tendon tenocytes express IL-1 receptors, and IL-1β induces the expression of MMP-1, MMP-3, and MMP-13 in tenocytes without altering the levels of TIMP-1 or TIMP-2 mRNA [74]. This suggests that IL-1β shifts the balance of MMPs and inhibitors in favor of tissue destruction.

MMP-14 is important for the physiologic activation of the inactive precursor form of MMP-2. The expression of MMP-2 can be up-regulated in Achilles tendinopathy [62], although Ireland et al [61] demonstrated no such up-regulation in tendinopathic Achilles tendon; however, they used autopsy materials as control tissue, whereas Alfredson et al [62] used clinically normal-looking tendon tissue in the same tendinopathic tendon. Also, interindividual variations could have generated the different results.

In another disorder of fibroblast proliferation and production of ECM, palmar fibromatosis (Dupuytren's contracture), MMP-2, MMP-14, and TIMP-2 are up-regulated [75]. This upregulation was present in the fibroblasts and endothelial cells of the palmar fascia of these patients. The genes for MMP-14 and types I and III collagen are also up-regulated in Achilles tendinopathy [61].

Physical exercise can influence local MMP and TIMP activities in the human Achilles tendon [76], with a pronounced increase in local levels of pro–MMP-9 after exercise. This study suggests that MMP-9 has a role in a potential inflammation reaction in human Achilles tendon that is induced by intensive exercise. Also, exercise causes a rapid increase in serum MMP-9 [77], probably as a result of increased leukocytes in the circulation [78]. Koskinen et al [76] also observed that the MMP-2 inhibitory activity of TIMP-1 and TIMP-2 increased in response to exercise.

Summary

MMPs may play a role in the pathogenesis of tendinopathy. MMPs can be up- or down-regulated, locally and systemically, in tendinopathy and complete tears of tendon. A balance exists between expression of MMPs and TIMPs to maintain tendon homeostasis. Table 2 highlights the main features of the role that is played by MMPs in the pathogenesis of tendinopathy. More research is required to determine the mechanism of action and regulation of MMPs in tendinopathy to promote the development of specific therapeutic strategies.

Table 2
Main roles of some matrix metalloproteases and tissue inhibitors of metalloproteases

MMP/TIMP	Main roles
MMP-1	Degrades type I collagen [73]
	Up-regulated in acute tendon tears [15]
	Up-regulated in tendinopathy [58,59]
	Up-regulated in response to shear stress [64]
	Down-regulated in response to cyclical strain and static tensile load [65,66]
MMP-2	Up-regulated in tendinopathy [62]
	May be up-regulated [57] or down-regulated [15] in complete tendon tears
	Inhibits TIMP-1 and TIMP-2 in response to exercise [76]
MMP-3	Plays a major role in maintenance and remodelling of normal tendon [15,61]
	Down-regulated in tendinopathy and complete tendon tears [15,60,61,62]
	Up-regulated in response to shear force [64]
MMP-13	Up-regulated in complete tendon tears [60]
MMP-9	Up-regulated following exercise [76,77]
TIMP-1	Down-regulated in tendinopathy [58,59,61]
	Up-regulated transiently following an acute tendon tear [57]
	Inhibits excessive degeneration of ECM by MMP-2 [57]
TIMP-2	Down-regulated in tendinopathy [61] and complete tendon tears [60]
TIMP-3	
TIMP-4	

References

[1] Bestwick CS, Maffulli N. Reactive oxygen species and tendon problems: review and Hypothesis. Sports Med Arthroscopy Rev 2000;8:6–16.

[2] Kastelic J, Galeski A, Baer E. The multicomposite structure of tendon. Connect Tissue Res 1978;6:11–23.

[3] Józsa L, Kannus P. Structure and metabolism of normal tendons. In: Józsa L, Kannus P, editors. Human tendons: anatomy, physiology and pathology. Champaign (IL): Human Kinetics; 1997. p. 46–95.

[4] Józsa L, Kannus P, Balint JB, et al. Three dimensional ultrastructure of human tendons. Acta Anat (Basel) 1991;142:306–12.

[5] Ochiai N, Matsui T, Miyaji N, et al. Vascular anatomy of flexor tendons. I. Vincular system and blood supply of the profundus tendon in the digital sheath. J Hand Surg [Am] 1979;4:321–30.

[6] Aumailley M, Gayraud B. Structure and biological activity of the extracellular matrix. J Mol Med 1998;76:253–65.

[7] Maffulli N, Barrass V, Ewen SW. Light microscopic histology of Achilles tendon ruptures. A comparison with unruptured tendons. Am J Sports Med 2000;28(6):857–63.

[8] Viidik A. Tensile strength: properties of Achilles tendon systems in trained and untrained rabbits. Acta Orthop Scand 1969;40:261–72.

[9] Williams IF. Cellular and biochemical composition of healing tendons. In: Jenkins DHR, editor. Ligament injuries and their treatment. London: Chapman and Hall; 1985. p. 43–57.

[10] Riley G. The pathogenesis of tendinopathy. A molecular prospective. Rheumatol 2004;43: 131–42.

[11] Movin T, Gad A, Reinholt FP, et al. Tendon pathology in long-standing achillodynia—biopsy findings in 40 patients. Acta Orthop Scand 1997;68(2):170–5.

[12] Rolf C, Movin T. Etiology, histopathology and outcome of surgery in achillodynia. Foot Ankle Int 1997;18(9):565–9.

[13] Tallon C, Maffulli N, Ewen SW. Ruptured Achilles tendons are significantly more degenerated than tendinopathic tendons. Med Sci Sports Exerc 2001;33(12):1983–90.

[14] Aström M, Rausing A. Chronic Achilles tendinopathy. A survey of surgical and histopathological findings. Clin Orthop 1995;316:151–64.

[15] Riley GP, Curry V, DeGroot J, et al. Matrix metalloproteinase activities and their relationship with collagen remodelling in tendon pathology. Matrix Biol 2002;21:185–95.

[16] Corps AN, Harrall RL, Curry VA, et al. Ciprofloxacin enhances the stimulation of matrix metalloproteinase 3 expression by interlukin-1 beta in human tendon-derived cells. A potential mechanism of fluoroquinolone-induced tendinopathy. Arthritis Rheum 2002;46:3034–40.

[17] Corps AN, Curry VA, Harrall RL, et al. Ciprofloxacin reduces the stimulation of prostaglandin E2 output by interleukin-1β in human tendon-derived cells. Rheumatol 2003;42:1306–10.

[18] Pierfitte C, Royer RJ. Tendon disorders with fluoroquinolones. Therapie 1996;51:419–20.

[19] Birkedal-Hansen H, Moore WGI, Bodden MK, et al. Matrix metalloproteinase: a review. Crit Rev Oral Biol Med 1993;4:197–250.

[20] Oblander SA, Somerville RPT, Apte SS. An update on metalloproteinases in the musculoskeletal system. Curr Opin Orthop 2003;14:322–8.

[21] Cawston TE, Billlington C. Metalloproteinases in rheumatic diseases. J Pathol 1996;180:115–7.

[22] Saarialho-Kere UK, Vaalamo M, Airola K, et al. Interstitial collagenase is expressed by keratinocytes that are actively involved in re-epithilialization in blistering skin diseases. J Invest Derm 1995;104:982–8.

[23] Eriksen EF. Normal and pathological remodelling of human trabecular bone: three dimensional reconstruction of the remodelling sequence in normals and in metabolic bone disease. Endocr Rev 1986;7:379–408.

[24] Werb Z, Alexander CM, Adler RR. Expression and function of matrix metalloproteinases in development. In: Birkedal-Hansen H, Werb Z, Welgus HG, et al, editors. Matrix metalloproteinases and inhibitors. Stuttgart (Germany): Gustav Fischer; 1992. p. 337–43.

[25] Goldberg GI, Eisen AZ. Extracellular matrix metalloproteinases in tumor invasion and metastasis. Cancer Treat Res 1991;53:421–40.

[26] Johannsson N, Airola K, Grenman R, et al. Expression of collagenase-3 (MMP-13) in squamous cell carcinoma of the head and neck. Am J Pathol 1997;151:499–508.

[27] Matrisian LM, McDonnell S, Miller DB, et al. The role of matrix metalloproteinase stromelysin in the progression of squamous cell carcinomas. Am J Med Sci 1991;302:157–62.

[28] Mignatti P, Rifkin DB. Biology and biochemistry of proteinases in tumor invasion. Physiol Rev 1993;73:161–95.

[29] Tryggvason K, Hoyhtya M, Pyke C. Type IV collagenases in invasive tumors. Breast Cancer Res Treat 1993;24:209–18.

[30] Chandler S, Miller KM, Clements JM, et al. Matrix metalloproteinases, tumor necrosis factor and multiple sclerosis: an overview. J Neuroimmunol 1997;72:155–61.

[31] Birkedal-Hansen H. Role of matrix metalloproteinases in periodontal diseases. J Periodontol 1993;64(5 Suppl):474–84.

[32] Meikle MC, Hembry RM, Holley J, et al. Immunolocalization of matrix metalloproteinases and TIMP-1 in human gingival tissues from periodontitis patients. J Periodontol Res 1994;29:118–26.

[33] Robert V, Besse S, Sabri A, et al. Differential regulation of matrix metalloproteinases associated with aging and hypertension in the rat heart. Lab Invest 1997;76:729–38.

[34] Brinckerhoff CE. Regulation of metalloproteinase gene expression: implication for osteoarthritis. Crit Rev Euk Gene Expr 1992;2:145–64.

[35] Enomoto H, Inoki I, Komiya K, et al. Vascular endothelial growth factor isoforms and their receptors are expressed in human osteoarthritic cartilage. Am J Pathol 2003;162:171–81.

[36] Firestein GS. Mechanisms of tissue destruction and cellular activation in rheumatoid arthritis. Curr Opin Rheumatol 1992;4:348–54.

[37] Salminen HJ, Saamanen AM, Vankemmelbeke MN, et al. Differential expression patterns of matrix metalloproteinases and their inhibitors during development of osteoarthritis in transgenic mouse model. Ann Rheum Dis 2002;61:591–7.

[38] Lin R, Amiuka N, Sasaki T, et al. 1 Alpha, 25-dihydroxyvitamin D3 promotes vascularization of the chondroosseous junction by stimulating expression of vascular endothelial growth factor and matrix metalloproteinase 9. J Bone Miner Res 2002;17:1604–12.

[39] Testa V, Capasso G, Maffulli N, et al. Proteases and antiproteases in cartilage homeostasis. Clin Orthop Rel Res 1994;308:79–84.

[40] Tetlow LC, Woolley DE. Histamine stimulates matrix metalloproteinase-3 and 13 production by human articular chondrocytes in vitro. Ann Rheum Dis 2002;61:737–40.

[41] Yasuda T, Poole AR, Shimizu M, et al. Involvement of CD44 in induction of matrix metalloproteinases by a COOH-terminal heparin-binding fragment of fibronectin in human articular cartilage in culture. Arthritis Rheum 2003;48(5):1271–80.

[42] Gomez DE, Alonso DF, Yoshiji H, et al. Tissue inhibitors of metalloproteinases: structure, regulation and biological functions. Eur J Cell Biol 1997;74:111–22.

[43] Goupille P, Jayson MIV, Valat J, et al. Matrix metalloproteinases: the clue to intervertebral disc degeneration? Spine 1998;23(14):1612–26.

[44] Dalton S, Cawston TE, Riley GP, et al. Human shoulder tendon biopsy samples in organ culture produce procollagenase and tissue inhibitor of metalloproteinases. Ann Rheum Dis 1995;54(7):571–7.

[45] Dayer JM, Burger D. Interleukin-1, tumor necrosis factor and their specific inhibitors. Eur Cytokine Netw 1994;5:563–71.

[46] Dayer JM, Arend WP. Cytokines and growth factors. In: Kelly WN, Harris Jr ED, Ruddy S, et al, editors. Textbook of rheumatology. Philadelphia: WB Saunders; 1997. p. 267–86.

[47] Mauviel A. Cytokine regulation of metalloproteinase gene expression. J Cell Biochem 1993;53:288–95.

[48] Wright JK, Cawston TE, Hazleman BL. Transforming growth factor β stimulates the production of the tissue inhibitor of metalloproteinase by human synovial and skin fibroblasts. Biochem Biophys Acta 1991;1094:207–10.

[49] Lotz M, Gurene PA. Interleukin-6 induces the synthesis of tissue inhibitor of metalloproteinase-1/ erythroid potentiating activity (TIMP-1/EPA). J Biol Chem 1991;266:2017–20.

[50] Kahari VM, Saarialho-Kere U. Matrix metalloproteinases in skin. Exp Dermatol 1997;6: 199–213.

[51] Nagase H, Woessner JF. Matrix metalloproteinases. J Biol Chem 1999;274:21491–4.

[52] Ravanti L, Kahari VM. Matrix metalloproteinases in wound repair. Int J Mol Med 2000;6: 391–407.

[53] Vincenti MP. The matrix metalloproteinase (MMP) and tissue inhibitor of metalloproteinase (TIMP) genes. Transcriptional and posttranscriptional regulation, signal transduction and cell-type-specific expression. Methods Mol Biol 2001;151:121–47.

[54] Aimes RT, Quigley JP. Matrix metalloproteinase-2 is an interstitial collagenase. Inhibitor-free enzyme catalyses the cleavage of collagen fibrils and soluble native type I collagen generating the specific 3/4 and 1/4 length fragments. J Biol Chem 1995;270:5872–6.

[55] Konttinen YT, Ceponis A, Takagi M, et al. New collagenolytic enzymes/cascade identified at the pannus–hard tissue junction in rheumatoid arthritis; destruction from above. Matrix Biol 1998; 17:585–601.

[56] Shlopov BV, Lie WR, Mainardi CL, et al. Osteoarthritic lesions—involvement of three different collagenases. Arthr Rheum 1997;40:2065–74.

[57] Choi HR, Seiji K, Kazuyoshi H, et al. Expression and enzymatic activity of MMP-2 during healing process of acute supraspinatus tendon tear in rabbits. J Orthop Res 2002;20:927–33.

[58] Fu SC, Chan BP, Wang W, et al. Increased expression of matrix metalloproteinase1 (MMP-1) in 11 patients with patellar tendinosis. Acta Orthop Scand 2002;73(6):658–62.

[59] Riley GP, Harrall RL, Cawston TE, et al. Interstitial collagenase (MMP-1), interleukin 1-α and tendon collagen degradation. Br J Rheumatol 1997;36:45.

[60] Lo IKY, Marchuk L, Hollinshead R, et al. Matrix metalloproteinase and tissue inhibitor of matrix metalloproteinase mRNA levels are specifically altered in torn rotator cuff tendons. Am J Sports Med 2004;32(5):1223–9.

[61] Ireland D, Harrall R, Curry V, et al. Multiple changes in gene expression in chronic human Achilles tendinopathy. Matrix Biol 2001;20:159–69.

[62] Alfredson H, Lorentzon M, Bäckman S, et al. cDNA- arrays and real time quantitative PCR techniques in the investigation of chronic Achilles tendinosis. J Orthop Res 2003;21:970–5.

[63] Buttice G, Duterque-Coquillaud M, Basuyaux JP, et al. Erg, an Ets-family member, differentially regulates human collagenase 1 (MMP-1) and stromelysin 1 (MMP-3) gene expression by physi-cally interacting with the Fos/Jun complex. Oncogene 1996;13:2297–306.

[64] Archambault JM, Elfervig-Wall MK, Tsuzaki M, et al. Rabbit tendon cells produce MMP-3 in response to fluid flow without significant calcium transients. J Biomech 2002;35:303–9.

[65] Lavagnino M, Arnoczky SP, Tian T, et al. Effect of amplitude and frequency of cyclic tensile strain on the inhibition of MMP-1 mRNA expression in tendon cells: an in vitro study. Connect Tissue Res 2003;44:181–7.

[66] Amoczky SP, Tian T, Lavagnino M, et al. In situ tensile load modulates inhibition of MMP-1 expression in rat tail tendon cells in a dose-dependant manner through a cytoskeletally-based based mechanotransduction mechanism. J Orthop Res 2004;22(2):328–33.

[67] Maffulli N, Ewen SW, Waterston SW, et al. Tenocytes from ruptured and tendinopathic Achilles tendons produce greater quantities of type-III collagen than tenocytes from normal tendons. An in vitro model of human tendon healing. Am J Sports Med 2000;28:499–505.

[68] Riley GP, Harrall RL, Constant CR, et al. Tendon degeneration and chronic shoulder pain: changes in the collagen composition of human rotator cuff tendons in rotator cuff tendinitis. Ann Rheum Dis 1994;53:359–66.

[69] Chard MD, Cawston TE, Riley GP, et al. Rotator cuff degeneration and lateral epicondylitis—a comparative histological study. Ann Rheum Dis 1994;5:30–4.

[70] Riley GP, Goddard MJ, Hazleman BL. Histopathological assessment and pathological sig-nificance of matrix degeneration in supraspinatus tendons. Rheumatol 2001;40:229–30.

[71] Blevins FT, Djurasovic M, Flatow EL, et al. Biology of the rotator cuff tendon. Orthop Clin N Am 1997;28:1–16.

[72] Fan L, Sarkar K, Franks DJ, et al. Estimation of total collagen and types I and III collagen in canine rotator cuff tendons. Calcif Tissue Int 1997;61:223–9.

[73] Knauper V, Lopez-Otin C, Smith B, et al. Biochemical characterization of human collagenase-3. J Biol Chem 1996;271:1544–50.

[74] Tsuzaki M, Guyton G, Garrett W, et al. IL-1 beta induces COX2, MMP-1, -3 and -13, ADAMTS-4, IL-1 beta and IL-6 in human tendon cells. J Orthop Res 2003;21:256–64.

[75] Roebuck MM, Sathyamoorthy P, Kalogrianitis S, et al. Effects of tourniquet ischaemia on HIF-1α and MMP-9 production by tissue from palmer fascia. Int J Exp Pathol 2003;84(4): A17–8.

[76] Koskinen SOA, Heinemeier KM, Olesen JL, et al. Physical exercise can influence the levels of matrix metalloproteinases and their inhibitors in tendon related connective tissue. J Appl Physiol 2004;96:861–4.

[77] Koskinen SOA, Höyhtyä M, Turpeemnniemi-Hujanen T, et al. Serum concentrations of collagen-degrading enzymes and their inhibitors after downhill running. Scand J Med Sci Sports 2001;11:9–15.

[78] McCarthy DA, Dale MM. The leucocytosis of exercise. A review and model. Sports Med 1988;6:333–63.

ELSEVIER
SAUNDERS

Foot Ankle Clin N Am
10 (2005) 279–292

FOOT AND
ANKLE CLINICS

Paratendinopathy

Mika Paavola, MD, PhD[a,b,*], Tero A.H. Järvinen[b,c,d]

[a]Department of Orthopaedics and Traumatology, Helsinki University Central Hospital,
Töölö Hospital, Helsinki, Finland
[b]Department of Orthopaedic Surgery, Medical School and the Institute of Medical Technology,
University of Tampere, Tampere, Finland
[c]Department of Surgery, Tampere University Hospital, Tampere, Finland
[d]The Burnham Institute, 10901 North Torrey Pines Road, La Jolla, CA 92037, USA

Competitive and recreational sports have become an important part of life in Western countries over the last 4 decades. Competitive and professional sports have received much attention in the mass media, which, in turn, has increased the demands on athletes. This development has been followed by the increased prevalence of sport injuries, especially overuse injuries, because athletes are required to train more intensely and for longer. This is reflected by the dramatic increase in overuse injuries on the Achilles tendon [1–6]. Achilles tendon problems are not restricted to competitive athletes, but also affect recreational sports participants as well as individuals in occupations where the lower limbs are under excessive strains [1–6].

The spectrum of Achilles tendon disorders and overuse injuries ranges from inflammation of the peritendinous tissue (peritendinitis, paratendinopathy), structural degeneration of the tendon (tendinosis), insertional disorders (retrocalcanear bursitis and insertional tendinopathy) to tendon rupture [1,2,4,7]. The most common symptom of the Achilles tendon overuse injury is the pain-induced limitation in sports and other physically demanding activities, whereas daily activities normally are not affected. The goal of management is to return patients to their

* Corresponding author. Department of Orthopedics and Traumatology, Helsinki University Central Hospital, Töölö Hospital, Helsinki, Finland.
  E-mail address: mika.paavola@uta.fi (M. Paavola).

1083-7515/05/$ – see front matter © 2005 Elsevier Inc. All rights reserved.
doi:10.1016/j.fcl.2005.01.008   *foot.theclinics.com*

desired level of physical activity without significant residual pain. In athletes, an additional demand is that the recovery time should be as short as possible.

Based on their location, Achilles tendon disorders can be grouped into injuries that occur at the myotendinous junction, in the main body of the tendon, or at the osteotendinous junction. There are no universally accepted criteria to consider an overuse tendon injury as acute or chronic [2]. El Hawary et al [8] suggested that when the symptoms have been experienced for less than 2 weeks, the Achilles disorder should be classified as acute tendinopathy; if the symptoms have been experienced for 2 to 6 weeks, it should be classified as subacute tendinopathy; and if the symptoms have persisted for longer than 6 weeks, it should be classified as chronic tendinopathy. These arbitrary distinctions are not based on histopathology findings or clinical outcome criteria. Nevertheless, they provide a descriptive framework for the condition.

The terminology that is used in the literature for the painful conditions of the Achilles tendon is confusing, and most often, does not reflect the pathology of the tendon disorder. Terms, such as "tendinitis," "tenonitis," and "tendonitis" have been used widely to describe this disorder, although inflammatory cell infiltration or markers of the inflammatory process are not seen in the tendon tissue biopsies of chronic Achilles tendon problems [1,9–12]. The terms "tendinopathy," "tenopathy," "tendinosis," "partial rupture," "paratenonitis," "tenosynovitis," "tendovaginitis," "peritendinitis," and "achillodynia" have been used to describe the noninsertional overuse problems of tendons. Åström [13] preferred the term "achillodynia" as a symptomatic diagnosis, and recommended "tendinosis" and "peritendinitis" be reserved for cases where the pathology was verified by surgical exploration or by histologic biopsies. Maffulli et al [14] proposed that a combination of pain, swelling, and impaired performance should be given the clinical label of "tendinopathy." We use the term "Achilles paratendinopathy" in clinical practice to describe activity-related Achilles tendon pain combined with tenderness on palpation, swelling around the tendon, and no intratendinous pathology on the basis of patient history, clinical examination, or imaging [9,14]. The necessity to differentiate Achilles paratendinopathy from tendinopathy, from histopathologic and clinical aspects, is uncertain, however, because no studies have compared the outcome of these two conditions.

Anatomy and function of the paratendinous structures of the Achilles tendon

The Achilles tendon constitutes the distal insertion of the gastrocnemius–soleus musculotendinous unit (ie, the triceps surae muscle) [2,3]. The Achilles tendon is surrounded throughout its length by thin gliding membranes, the paratenon. The paratenon functions as an elastic sleeve (although probably not as effectively as a true tendon sheath), and permits free movement of the tendon within the surrounding tissues [1,15]. The paratenon forms a thin space between the tendon and the crural fascia, which is covered by subcutaneous fat and skin [15,16]. Under the paratenon, the entire Achilles tendon is surrounded by a fine, smooth, connective tissue sheath, the epitenon. On its outer surface, the epitenon is in contact with the paratenon. The inner surface of the epitenon is continuous with the endotenon, which binds the collagen fibers and fiber bundles together and provides the neural, vascular, and lymphatic supply to the tendon [1].

The paratenon is richly vascularized and it provides blood supply to the Achilles tendon itself [1,2,17,18]. The neural supply to the Achilles tendon and the surrounding paratenon is provided by nerves from the attaching muscles and by small fasciculi from cutaneous nerves, in particular the sural nerve [19]. The number of nerves and nerve endings is small, and many nerve fibers terminate on the tendon surface or in the paratenon [1]. These nerves follow the vascular channels within the long axis of the tendon, anastomose with each other by way of obliquely- and transversely-oriented fibers, and terminate in sensory nerve endings [1]. In patients who have Achilles tendon overuse injury, the sensory nerve endings follow the paratendinous neovascularization and may be a cause of Achilles tendon pain [20].

Epidemiology

The overall yearly incidence rate for running injuries varies between 24% and 65% [21,22]. Approximately 50% to 75% of all running injuries are overuse injuries from constant repetition of the same movement, mostly in the Achilles tendon and in the tendons that surround the knee joint [4]. The occurrence of Achilles tendon overuse injuries is greatest in athletes who participate in middle- and long-distance running, orienteering, track and field, tennis, and other ball games [4,6,23–29]; the annual incidence of Achilles tendon overuse injuries is between 7% and 9% in top-level runners [24,25]. The most common clinical diagnosis of Achilles overuse injuries is paratendinopathy or tendinopathy (55%–65%), followed by insertional problems (retrocalcanear bursitis and insertional tendinopathy) (20%–25%) [4,6,28,29].

In a cohort study with an 11-year follow up, questionnaire-reported Achilles tendon overuse injuries were present in 79 of 269 male orienteering runners (29%) and 7 of 188 controls (4%); the age-adjusted odds ratio was 10.0 in runners compared with controls [30].

Kvist [4,23] studied the epidemiologic factors associated with Achilles tendon injuries in a large group of sports patients. In 698 patients, 66% had paratendinopathy or tendinopathy, and 23% Achilles tendon insertional problems. In 8% of the patients, the injury was located at the myotendinous junction; 3% of all patients had a total tendon rupture. Of the patients who had Achilles tendon injury, 89% were men. Running was the main sporting activity of patients who had Achilles tendon injury (53%), whereas patients who participated in running sports accounted for 27% of all patients who were studied in that clinic. Some form of malalignment of the lower extremity was found in 60% of patients who had Achilles tendon overuse injury.

Etiology and pathophysiology

The etiology of Achilles tendon overuse injuries is multi-factorial [28,31]. Training errors have been reported with 60% to 70% of the running injuries [25,32]. The most common of these include running too long a distance, running at too great an intensity, increasing distance too greatly or intensity too rapidly, and performing too much uphill or downhill work [4,24,31]. Monotonous, asymmetric, and specialized training, such as running only (ie, without cross-training), as well as poor technique and fatigue are further risk factors for Achilles tendon overuse injuries [31]. Poor environmental conditions, such as cold weather, hard ground surface and slippery/icy surface, also have been suggested to promote Achilles tendon problems [32–34].

In the epidemiologic studies, various malalignment and biomechanical faults are claimed to play a causative role in two thirds of the athletes who had Achilles tendon disorders [4,6,23]; however, the mechanism by which this occurs remains controversial [35]. The most common, and perhaps most important, malalignment in the ankle that is associated with Achilles tendon overuse injury is hyperpronation of the foot [35]. Limited subtalar joint mobility and decreased range of motion of the ankle were more frequent in athletes who had Achilles tendinopathy than in those who had other complaints [23]. In addition, forefoot varus correlates with Achilles tendinopathy [4,23,35,36]. Recently, Kaufman et al [37] observed that increased hindfoot inversion and decreased ankle dorsiflexion with the knee in extension was associated with Achilles tendinopathy [37].

In addition to hyperpronation and the other aforementioned malalignments, leg length discrepancy is one of the more controversial potential contributing factors [31]. The traditional orthopedic view is that discrepancies of less than 20 mm are not clinically important [31]. In elite athletes, however, a discrepancy of more than 5 mm may be symptomatic and, consequently, for a discrepancy of 10 mm or more, a built-up shoe or shoe insert has been recommended to prevent overuse symptoms [31]. The true occurrence of these proposed biomechanical alterations, their magnitude and, above all, their clinical importance is unknown [31].

The importance of muscle weakness, muscle imbalance, and impaired musculotendinous flexibility in the development of Achilles tendon disorders also are debated. Muscular strength, power, endurance, and flexibility are an important part of physical performance, however, and, thus, can be important in the prevention of certain sports injuries, particularly tendon injuries [31]. If the muscle is weak or fatigued, the energy-absorbing capacity of the muscle–tendon unit is reduced and the muscle no longer protects the tendon from strain injury and subsequent pain [31]. Recently, good short-term improvements were reported in chronic Achilles tendinopathy with heavy-load eccentric training, a rehabilitation program that is based on increasing the length, tensile strength, and force of the muscle–tendon unit [38–42].

Pain is the most irritating symptom of Achilles tendon disorders. Traditionally, the pain associated with chronic Achilles paratendinopathy has been proposed to arise as a result of inflammation, separation of the collagen fibers, or tissue degeneration [43]. None of these hypotheses passes scientific scrutiny, however; many chronically painful Achilles tendons have no evidence of inflammation, and, conversely, many degenerated tendons do not cause pain [10,11,43]. Based on these observations, alternative explanations have been sought for the origin of pain in chronic tendon disorders. Preliminary clinical evidence was presented that the neovascularization of the paratenon and the accompanying nerves (ie, sensory nerve endings) could be responsible for the sensation of pain in the tendon region [44–46].

Histopathology of paratendinous alterations

In the acute phase of Achilles paratendinopathy, inflammatory cell reaction, circulatory impairment, and edema formation occur [1,2]. Crepitus, due to movement of the Achilles tendon within a paratenon that is filled with fibrin exudate, may be present. If the physiologic healing process fails or is delayed, the fibrin may organize and form adhesions that prohibit the normal gliding between the tendon, paratenon, and crural fascia [4,23]. In chronic Achilles paratendinopathy, the paratenon tissue becomes thickened as a result of fibrinous exudate; prominent and widespread proliferation of fibroblasts; formation of new connective tissue; and adhesions between tendon, paratenon, and crural fascia [47–50].

Normal fibroblasts and myofibroblasts have been identified in the paratenon of patients who had chronic Achilles paratendinopathy [46]. If heavy mechanical strains are imposed on the tendon, the fibroblasts secrete transforming growth factor–β, which, in turn, acts in an auto- or paracrine manner on tenocytes, which acquire a myofibroblast phenotype [51,52]. Myofibroblasts have cytoplasm fibers of α–smooth muscle actin, and are thus capable of producing the forces that are required in physiologic processes as granulation contraction in different tissues [51,52]. In Achilles paratendinopathy, myofibroblasts are especially present at the sites of scar formation [46], and myofibroblasts constitute approximately 20% of peritendinous cells in chronic paratendinopathy [45]. Myofibroblasts synthesize abundant collagen I and III [47,48], and are probably responsible for the formation of permanent scarring and the shrinkage of peritendinous tissue around the tendon [46,50]. These cells also most likely play an important role in the clinical symptoms, because they can induce and maintain a prolonged contracted state in the peritendinous adhesions around the tendon [46,50]. This may lead to constriction of vascular channels and to impaired circulation and further contribute to the pathogenesis of Achilles tendinopathy [46,50]. The proliferating connective tissue around the Achilles tendon causes increased intratendinous tension and pressure, and results in increased friction between the tendon, paratenon, crural fascia, and the overlying skin [46,50].

Diagnosis of Achilles paratendinopathy

Pain is the cardinal symptom of Achilles paratendinopathy that leads a patient to seek medical attention. It can be used to classify the severity of the disorder [1]. In patients who have acute Achilles paratendinopathy, the tendon is diffusely swollen and, on palpation, tenderness usually is greatest in the middle third of the tendon. Sometimes, in the acute phase, crepitation can be appreciated at palpation [4,32]. Typically, in patients who have acute symptoms, the area of swelling and tenderness does not move when the ankle joint is dorsiflexed. Furthermore, areas of increased erythema, local heat, and palpable tendon nodules or defects also may be present at clinical examination. In addition, ankle instability and mal-alignment of the lower extremity, especially in the foot, should be sought in patients who have Achilles tendon complaints [1–3].

In chronic Achilles paratendinopathy, exercise-induced pain is the main symptom, whereas crepitation and swelling may well diminish [1–3]. A tender, nodular swelling usually indicates tendinopathy of the main body of the tendon [32,53], and these focal tender nodules move as the ankle is dorsiflexed and plantarflexed [54]. Differential diagnosis of Achilles tendon disorders is found in Table 1. There is a marked overlap of the findings in history and physical examination, and, in clinical practice, overuse injuries have features of more than one pathophysiologic entity (eg, patients who have tendinosis usually have additional peritendinous pathology). In most cases, however, an adequate history and physical examination should give the correct diagnosis.

Ultrasonography (US) is a reliable diagnostic method for Achilles paratendinopathy if adhesions can be seen around an Achilles tendon [55]; however, US may fail to detect adhesions and produce false negative results in patients who have few adhesions [55]. In acute Achilles paratendinopathy, US reveals fluid surrounding the tendon [55], whereas paratendinous adhesions can be seen as thickening of the hypoechoic paratenon with poorly-defined borders in the chronic form of the disorder [56].

MRI has been used extensively to visualize tendon pathology [57,58]. The ability of MRI to acquire images from multiple planes (longitudinal, transverse, oblique) also is a clear advantage [2,58]. MRI is expensive and may not be widely available in some countries, and scanning may be time-consuming and slow. Also, there could be persistence of altered signal after surgery, with unclear correlation with the clinical picture [2]. In addition, the normal anatomy of an asymptomatic Achilles tendon may vary and cause diagnostic misinterpretation with MRI [59]. In patients who have pure chronic Achilles paratendinopathy

Table 1
Differential diagnosis of Achilles tendon disorders

	Paratendinopathy	Tendinosis	Partial rupture	Insertional disorder	Anomalous soleus	Complete rupture
History						
Pain on exertion	X	X	X	X	X	X
Pain only in tendon insertion				X		
Pain behind Achilles tendon					X	
Gradual onset of symptoms	X	X		X	X	
Sudden onset of symptoms			X			X
Stiffness and pain in the morning	X	X	X	X	X	
Clinical findings						
Tenderness in middle third of tendon	X	X	X		X	X
Tenderness of tendon insertion				X		
Swelling	X	X	X	X	X	X
Palpable nodules that do not move when ankle is dorsiflexed	X					
Palpable nodules move when ankle is dorsiflexed		X	X			
Swelling or bulbous mass at medial or lateral side of Achilles tendon					X	
Crepitation	X					
Palpable gap			X			X
Thompson test positive						X

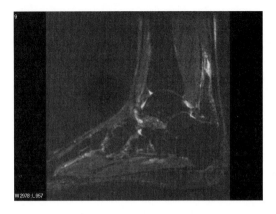

Fig. 1. Longitudinal T2-weighted MRI of the Achilles tendon with paratendinopathy (and additional tendinopathy). Paratendinous signal changes are seen ventrally 2 cm to 4 cm above the tendon insertion. (Courtesy of Martti Kiuru, MD, PhD, Helsinki, Finland.)

(without tendinopathy of the main body of the Achilles tendon), MRI infrequently reveals any pathologic changes around the tendon (Fig. 1).

Management of Achilles paratendinopathy

Little reliable experimental or clinical scientific work has been performed on the pathophysiology, etiology, natural course, and management of Achilles tendon overuse injuries [2,3]. Without scientific backing and a firm understanding of the nature of tendon injuries and other tendon disorders, it is difficult to prescribe a proper management regimen for Achilles tendon problems. Conservative and surgical regimens vary considerably among countries, clinics, and physicians. Most management regimens are based only on what seemed to work empirically, without much scientific support [1–3].

In early Achilles paratendinopathy, various forms of conservative management are used [2,60]. Initial nonoperative management aims to identify and correct the above described predisposing factors of the chronic Achilles tendon problems [60]. Orthotics are used to correct malalignments and the training program is modified to place less strain on the Achilles tendon; if the symptoms are severe, the lower extremity (or just the ankle joint) is rested completely for 48 to 72 hours [2]. Although the use of nonsteroidal anti-inflammatory drugs (NSAIDs) did not affect the outcome of Achilles tendinopathy positively in a randomized clinical trial [61], they often are used for early management of pain from Achilles paratendinopathy [60]. The use of corticosteroid injections around the Achilles tendon should not be liberal [60,62], and they only should be administered by experienced physicians [62].

Surgical management is recommended to those patients who do not respond adequately to 3 to 6 months of conservative management [4,7,16,63–70]. No prospective randomized studies that compared operative and conservative management of Achilles paratendinopathy have been published, however; most of our knowledge on management efficacy is based on clinical experience and descriptive studies [2,3].

Tallon et al [71] reviewed studies that reported surgical outcomes in the management of chronic Achilles tendinopathy or paratendinopathy. Methodology scores of the studies generally were low, which indicated the limitations of these studies. A negative correlation was found between reported success rates and overall methodology scores; however, the positive correlation between year of publication and overall methodology score suggests that the quality of studies is improving. In Achilles tendon paratendinopathy, many investigators recommend that, after longitudinal division of the crural fascia, the paratenon should be incised and any macroscopic adhesions should be excised [7,16,64–67]. In some studies, adhesions were found mainly between the Achilles tendon and paratenon [7,64], whereas others reported that the paratenon adhered mainly to the crural fascia, or even to the skin [16,72].

The few studies of an endoscopic-assisted surgical release of adhesions around the Achilles tendon showed promising preliminary results [73–75], and the endoscopic technique may reduce early postoperative morbidity (Fig. 2). No studies have compared different operative methods in the treatment of Achilles paratendinopathy, however.

In most studies, surgery for Achilles tendon overuse injury gave satisfactory results in 75% to 100% of patients; however, most of these reports were retrospective and only in a few were the results based on objective evaluations. In addition, the underlying pathology usually has been heterogenous [7,16,63–70]. In a report by Paavola et al [76], operative management of Achilles paratendinopathy with or without tendinopathy of the main body of the Achilles tendon resulted in good and acceptable short-term results using subjective, clinical,

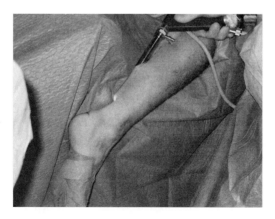

Fig. 2. Through aproximal portal incision, the scope is introduced below the crural fascia, which is released longitudinally. By way of endoscope, the adhesions are released with a retrograde knife blade or blunt dissector. (Courtesy of Martti Kiuru, MD, PhD, Helsinki, Finland.)

and functional tests as outcome criteria. A lower complication rate with operative management and a trend to better recovery was observed in patients who had pure paratendinous adhesions compared with those who had paratendinous adhesions combined with an intratendinous lesion [76].

An 11% overall complication rate was documented in a series of 432 consecutive patients [74]. In that study, most of the complications (54%) involved impaired skin wound healing [77].

Prognosis

Little is known about the natural course of Achilles paratendinopathy. An 8-year follow-up study [78] showed that the overall long-term prognosis of these patients was good. Seventy of the 83 patients (84%) were able to return to full levels of physical activity, and, at 8 years, 78 patients (94%) were asymptomatic or had only mild pain on strenuous exercise. Delays of up to 6 months between the onset of symptoms and initiation of conservative management did not compromise long-term outcome. Nevertheless, 24 of the 83 patients (29%) failed to respond to conservative management and underwent operative management. Also, even at the 8-year follow-up, there was a side-to-side difference between the involved and the uninvolved sides in the performance tests, clinical examination, and US findings. Furthermore, 41% of the patients developed some overuse symptoms (exertional pain with or without swelling and stiffness) also in the initially uninvolved Achilles tendon.

Summary

Because most Achilles tendon injuries take place in sports and there has been a general increase in the popularity of sporting activities, the number and incidence of Achilles tendon overuse injuries have increased in the industrialized countries during the last few decades. Clinically, overuse injuries of the Achilles tendon present as a combination of pain and swelling in the Achilles tendon region accompanied by impaired ability to perform strenuous activities. The term "Achilles paratendinopathy" is used in clinical practice to describe activity-related Achilles pain combined with tenderness on palpation, providing that there is no suspicion of intratendinous pathology on the basis of patient history, clinical examination, or imaging examinations.

Achilles tendinopathy is common in sports that require strenuous physical activities, such as running and jumping. The basic etiology of the Achilles tendinopathy is multi-factorial. Several extrinsic (eg, different training errors) and intrinsic factors (eg, hyperpronation) have been identified as predisposing to these problems.

In its acute phases, Achilles paratendinopathy often responds favorably to conservative management with rest or modified activity; cold; stretching; NSAIDs;, and correction of provoking, etiological factors. Surgical management is considered in patients who fail to respond to appropriate conservative management after 3 to 6 months. Operative management includes longitudinal division of the crural fascia and excision of the macroscopic fibrous adhesions between the paratenon, crural fascia, and the tendon.

Long-term prognosis of the Achilles paratendinopathy is good; approximately 80% of patients return to preinjury activity levels; however, almost 30% of patients require surgery. Patients who have unilateral Achilles tendinopathy have a high risk of sustaining Achilles tendinopathy in the uninvolved leg; almost half of patients who have Achilles tendinopathy develop symptoms in the contralateral leg over the years.

Acknowledgments

This work was supported by grants from the Sigrid Juselius Foundation, Helsinki, Finland; Tampere University Hospital Research Fund; the Research Council for Physical Education and Sport Ministry of Education, Finland; and the AO Foundation, Switzerland.

We would like to thank Professor Nicola Maffulli, Keele University School of Medicine, England, for the constructive criticism given. We also would like to thank Martti Kiuru, MD, PhD, Töölön sairaala, Helsinki, Finland, for providing the images that are used in this article.

References

[1] Jozsa L, Kannus P. Human tendons: anatomy, physiology, and pathology. Champaign (IL): Human Kinetics; 1997.

[2] Paavola M, Kannus P, Järvinen TAH, et al. Achilles tendinopathy. J Bone Joint Surg 2002; 84-A(11):2062–76.

[3] Maffulli N, Kader D. Tendinopathy of tendo Achillis. J Bone Joint Surg 2002;84-B(1):1–8.

[4] Kvist M. Achilles tendon injuries in athletes. Sports Med 1994;18:173–201.

[5] Kannus P, Jozsa L. Histopathological changes preceding spontaneous rupture of a tendon. A controlled study of 891 patients. J Bone Joint Surg 1991;73-A:1507–25.

[6] Järvinen TAH, Kannus P, Khan K, et al. Achilles tendon disorders—aetiology and epidemiology. Foot Ankle Clin, in press.

[7] Schepsis AA, Leach RE. Surgical management of Achilles tendinitis. Am J Sports Med 1987; 15:308–14.

[8] El Hawary R, Stanish WD, Curwin SL. Rehabilitation of tendon injuries in sport. Sports Med 1997;24:347–58.

[9] Khan KM, Cook JL, Kannus P, et al. Time to abandon the "tendinitis" myth. BMJ 2002; 324:626–7.

[10] Alfredson H, Thorsen K, Lorenzon R. In situ microdialysis in tendon tissue: high levels of glutamate, but not prostaglandin E_2 in chronic Achilles tendon pain. Knee Surg Sports Traumatol Arthrosc 1999;7:378–81.

[11] Alfredson H, Lorentzon M, Backman S, et al. cDNA-arrays and real-time quantitative PCR techniques in the investigation of chronic Achilles tendinosis. J Orthop Res 2003;21(6):970–5.

[12] Kannus P, Järvinen TLN, Järvinen TAH, et al. Painful Achilles tendon and its treatment. Scand J Med Sci Sports 2004;14(2):69–71.

[13] Åström M. On the nature and etiology of chronic Achilles tendinopathy [master's thesis]. Malmö (Sweden): Lund University; 1997.

[14] Maffulli N, Khan KM, Puddu G. Overuse tendon conditions: time to change a confusing terminology. Arthroscopy 1998;14:840–3.

[15] Perry JR. Achilles tendon anatomy: Normal and pathologic. Foot Ankle Clin 1997;2:363–70.

[16] Kvist H, Kvist M. The operative treatment of chronic calcaneal paratenonitis. J Bone Joint Surg 1980;62-B:353–7.

[17] Carr AJ, Norris SH. The blood supply of the calcaneal tendon. J Bone Joint Surg 1989;71-B: 100–1.

[18] Kvist M, Hurme T, Kannus P, et al. Vascular density at the myotendinous junction of the rat gastrocnemius muscle after immobilization and remobilization. Am J Sports Med 1995;23: 359–64.

[19] Stilwell DL. The innervation of tendons and aponeuroses. Am J Anat 1957;100:289–317.

[20] Alfredson H, Öhberg L, Forsgren S. Is vasculo-neural ingrowth the cause of pain in chronic Achilles tendinosis? An investigation using ultrasonography and colour Doppler, immunohistochemistry, and diagnostic injections. Knee Surg Sports Traumatol 2003;11:334–8.

[21] Hoeberigs JH. Factors related to the incidence of running injuries. A review. Sports Med 1992; 13:408–22.

[22] Van Mechelen W. Running injuries. A review of the epidemiological literature. Sports Med 1992;14:320–35.

[23] Kvist M. Achilles tendon injuries in athletes. Ann Chir Gynaecol 1991;80:188–201.

[24] Leppilahti J, Orava S, Karpakka J, et al. Overuse injuries of the Achilles tendon. Ann Chir Gynaecol 1991;80:202–7.

[25] Johansson C. Injuries in elite orienteers. Am J Sports Med 1986;14:410–5.

[26] Lysholm J, Wiklander J. Injuries in runners. Am J Sports Med 1987;15:168–71.

[27] Fahlström M, Lorentzon R, Alfredson H. Painful conditions in the Achilles tendon region in elite badminton players. Am J Sports Med 2002;30:51–4.

[28] Järvinen TAH, Kannus P, Józsa L, et al. Achilles tendon injuries. Curr Opin Rheumatol 2001; 13(2):150–5.

[29] Järvinen M. Epidemiology of tendon injuries in sports. Clin Sports Med 1992;11(3):493–504.

[30] Kujala UM, Sarna S, Kaprio J, et al. Heart attacks and lower-limb function in master endurance athletes. Med Sci Sports Exerc 1999;31:1041–6.

[31] Kannus P. Etiology and pathophysiology of chronic tendon disorders in sports. Scand J Sports Med 1997;7(2):78–85.

[32] James SL, Bates BT, Osterning LR. Injuries to runners. Am J Sports Med 1978;6:40–50.

[33] Hess GP, Capiello WL, Poole RM, et al. Prevention and treatment of overuse tendon injuries. Sports Med 1989;8:371–84.

[34] Milgrom C, Finestone A, Zin D, et al. Cold weather training: a risk factor for Achilles paratendinitis among recruits. Foot Ankle Int 2003;24(5):398–401.

[35] Nigg BM. The role of impact forces and foot pronation: A new paradigm. Clin J Sports Med 2001;11:2–9.

[36] McCrory JL, Martin DF, Lowery RB, et al. Etiologic factors associated with Achilles tendinitis in runners. Med Sci Sports Exerc 1999;31:1374–81.

[37] Kaufman KR, Brodine SK, Shaffer RA, et al. The effect of foot structure and range of motion on musculoskeletal overuse injuries. Am J Sports Med 1999;27:585–93.

[38] Alfredson H, Pietilä T, Jonsson P, et al. Heavy-load eccentric calf muscle training for the treatment of chronic Achilles tendinosis. Am J Sports Med 1998;26:360–6.

[39] Fahlström M, Jonsson P, Lorentzon R, et al. Chronic Achilles tendon pain treated with eccentric calf-muscle training. Knee Surg Sports Traumatol Arthrosc 2003;11(5):327–33.

[40] Öhberg L, Lorentzon R, Alfredson H. Eccentric training in patients with chronic Achilles tendinosis: normalised tendon structure and decreased thickness at follow up. Br J Sports Med 2004;38(1):8–11.

[41] Shalabi A, Kristoffersen-Wilberg M, Svensson L, et al. Eccentric training of the gastrocnemius-soleus complex in chronic Achilles tendinopathy results in decreased tendon volume and intratendinous signal as evaluated by MRI. Am J Sports Med 2004;32(5):1286–96.

[42] Roos EM, Engström M, Lagerquist A, et al. Clinical improvement after 6 weeks of eccentric exercise in patients with mid-portion Achilles tendinopathy—a randomized trial with 1-year follow-up. Scand J Med Sci Sports 2004;14(5):286–95.

[43] Khan KM, Cook JL, Maffulli N, et al. Where is the pain coming from in tendinopathy? It may be biochemical, not only structural, in origin. Br J Sports Med 2000;34:81–3.

[44] Alfredson H, Öhberg L, Forsgren S. Is vasculo-neural ingrowth the cause of pain in chronic Achilles tendinosis? An investigation using ultrasonography and colour Doppler, immunohistochemistry, and diagnostic injections. Knee Surg Sports Traumatol Arthrosc 2003;11(5):334–8.

[45] Öhberg L, Alfredson H. Sclerosing therapy in chronic Achilles tendon insertional pain—results of a pilot study. Knee Surg Spoorts Traumatol Arthrosc 2003;11(5):339–42.

[46] Öhberg L, Alfredson H. Ultrasound guided sclerosis of neovessels in painful chronic Achilles tendinosis: pilot study of a new treatment. Br J Sports Med 2002;36:173–5.

[47] Kvist M, Jozsa L, Järvinen M, et al. Fine structural alterations in chronic Achilles paratenonitis in athletes. Pathol Res Pract 1985;180(4):416–23.

[48] Kvist M, Jozsa L, Järvinen MJ, et al. Chronic Achilles paratenonitis in athletes: a histological and histochemical study. Pathol 1987;19:1–11.

[49] Kvist MH, Lehto MU, Jozsa L, et al. Chronic Achilles paratenonitis. An immunohistologic study of fibronectin and fibrinogen. Am J Sports Med 1988;16(6):616–23.

[50] Järvinen M, Józsa L, Kannus P, et al. Histopathological findings in chronic tendon disorders. Scand J Med Sci Sports 1997;7(2):86–95.

[51] Ehrlich HP, Desmouliere A, Diegelmann RF, et al. Morphological and immunochemical differences between keloid and hypertrophic scar. Am J Pathol 1994;145:105–13.

[52] Gabbiani G. The myofibroblast in wound healing and fibrocontractve diseases. J Pathol 2003;200:500–3.

[53] Galloway MT, Jokl P, Dayton OW. Achilles tendon overuse injuries. Clin Sports Med 1992;11:771–82.

[54] DiGiovanni BF, Gould JS. Achilles tendinitis and posterior heel disorders. Foot Ankle Clin 1997;2:411–28.

[55] Laine HR, Harjula ARJ, Peltokallio P. Ultrasonography as a differential diagnostic aid in achillodynia. J Ultrasound Med 1987;6:351–62.

[56] Paavola M, Paakkala T, Kannus P, et al. Ultrasonography in the differential diagnosis of Achilles tendon injuries and related disorders. A comparison between pre-operative ultrasonography and surgical findings. Acta Radiol 1998;39:612–9.

[57] Pope CF. Radiologic evaluation of tendons injuries. Clin Sports Med 1992;11:579–99.

[58] Kerr R, Forrester DM, Kingston S. Magnetic resonance imaging of foot and ankle trauma. Orthop Clin N Am 1990;21:591–601.

[59] Soila K, Karjalainen PT, Aronen HJ, et al. High resolution MR imaging of the asymptomatic Achilles tendon: new observations. Am J Roentgenol 1999;173:323–8.

[60] Sandmeier R, Renström PAFH. Diagnosis and treatment of chronic tendon disorders in sports. Scand J Med Sci Sports 1997;7(2):96–106.

[61] Åström M, Westlin N. No effect of piroxicam on achilles tendinopathy. A randomized study of 70 patients. Acta Orthop Scand 1992;63:631–4.

[62] Paavola M, Kannus P, Järvinen TAH, et al. Tendon healing: adverse role of steroid injection—myth or reality. Foot Ankle Clin 2002;7:501–13.

[63] Williams JGP. Achilles tendon lesions in sport. Sports Med 1986;3:114–35.

[64] Nelen G, Martens M, Burssens A. Surgical treatment of chronic Achilles tendinitis. Am J Sports Med 1989;17:754–9.

[65] Järvinen M. Lower leg overuse injuries in athletes. Knee Surg Sports Traumatol Arthrosc 1993;1(2):126–30.

[66] Leach RE, Schepsis AA, Takai H. Long-term results of surgical management of Achilles tendinitis in runners. Clin Orthop 1992;282:208–12.

[67] Lehto MUK, Järvinen M, Suominen P. Chronic Achilles peritendinitis and retrocalcanear bursitis. Long-term follow-up of surgically treated cases. Knee Surg Sports Traumatol Arthrosc 1994;2:182–5.

[68] Leppilahti J, Karpakka J, Gorra A, et al. Surgical treatment of overuse injuries to the Achilles tendon. Clin J Sport Med 1994;4:100–7.

[69] Schepsis AA, Wagner C, Leach RE. Surgical management of Achilles tendon overuse injuries. Am J Sports Med 1994;22:611–9.

[70] Schepsis AA, Jones H, Haas AL. Achilles tendon disorders in athletes. Am J Sports Med 2002;30(2):287–305.

[71] Tallon C, Coleman BD, Khan KM, et al. Outcome of surgery for chronic Achilles tendinopathy. A critical review. Am J Sports Med 2001;29:315–20.

[72] Rolf C, Movin T. Etiology, histology and outcome of surgery in achillodynia. Foot Ankle 1997;18:565–9.

[73] Van Dijk CN, Scholten PE, Kort NP. Tendoscopy (tendon heath endoscopy) for overuse tendon injuries. Operative Techniques Sports Med 1997;5:170–8.

[74] Maquirriain J, Ayerza M, Costa-Paz M, et al. Endoscopic surgery in chronic Achilles tendinopathies: a preliminary report. Arthroscopy 2002;18:298–303.

[75] Morag G, Maman E, Arbel R. Endoscopic treatment of hindfoot pathology. Arthroscopy 2003;19:E13.

[76] Paavola M, Kannus P, Orava S, et al. Surgical treatment for chronic Achilles tendinopathy. A prospective 7-month follow-up study. Br J Sports Med 2002;36:178–82.

[77] Paavola M, Orava S, Leppilahti J, et al. Complications after surgical treatment of a chronic Achilles tendon overuse injury. An analysis of 432 consecutive patients. Am J Sports Med 2000; 28:77–82.

[78] Paavola M, Kannus P, Paakkala T, et al. Long-term prognosis of patients with Achilles tendinopathy. An observational 8-year follow-up study. Am J Sports Med 2000;28:634–42.

ELSEVIER
SAUNDERS

Foot Ankle Clin N Am
10 (2005) 293–308

FOOT AND
ANKLE CLINICS

Tendinopathy of the Main Body of the Achilles Tendon

Anand M. Vora, MD[a], Mark S. Myerson, MD[b],*,
Francesco Oliva, MD[c],
Nicola Maffulli, MD, MS, PhD, FRCS(Orth)[c]

[a]Lake Forest Orthopaedic Associates, Illinois Bone & Joint Institute Ltd., 720 Florsheim Drive,
Libertyville, IL 60048, USA
[b]Institute for Foot and Ankle at Mercy, Mercy Medical Center, 301 St. Paul Place,
Baltimore, MD 21202, USA
[c]Department of Trauma and Orthopaedic Surgery, Keele University School of Medicine,
North Staffordshire Hospital, Thornburrow Drive, Hartshill, Stoke-on-Trent,
Staffordshire, ST4 7QB, UK

Achilles tendon disorders are common in athletes and within the general population [1,2]. Within the spectrum of Achilles tendon disorders, many different pathologic conditions exist. These conditions may coexist or may occur in isolation; the descriptive terminology used to describe the specific disorders of the Achilles tendon may be confusing and inaccurate. This article reviews chronic tendinopathy of the main body of the Achilles tendon [2], a condition with a combination of tendon pain, swelling, and impaired performance ability. Chronic tendinopathy has been described arbitrarily as the above condition with symptoms that last longer than 6 weeks [3]. The etiology, pathogenesis, anatomy, epidemiology, and natural history of chronic Achilles tendinopathy largely is unknown. Overuse injuries, poor vascularity, genetic makeup, gender, and endocrine or metabolic factors have been cited as possible etiologic factors [2,4].

Excessive loading of the Achilles tendon during athletic activities and work is regarded as the main pathologic stimulus that leads to tendinopathy [5], pos-

* Corresponding author.
E-mail address: mark4feet@aol.com (M.S. Myerson).

sibly as a result of imbalance between muscle power and tendon elasticity. The Achilles tendon may respond to repetitive supraphysiologic overload by inflammation of its sheath, degeneration of its body, or a combination of both [6]. Intensive eccentric repetitive loading of the Achilles tendon may affect collagen cross-linking, extracellular tendon matrix, and vascularity.

Achilles tendinopathy is statistically associated with a variety of intrinsic and extrinsic factors. Tendon vascularity, gastrocnemius–soleus dysfunction, age, gender, body weight and height, pes cavus deformity, and lateral ankle instability are common intrinsic factors. Changes in training pattern, poor technique, inadequate warm-up and stretching before training, previous injuries, footwear, and environmental factors (eg, training on hard, slippery, or slanting surfaces) are extrinsic factors [4–7].

Clinical aspects

A detailed history helps to identify the onset and possible contributing factors in a painful Achilles tendon. The duration of pain and its relationship to various activities should be documented. The clinical grading of the pain that is associated with tendinopathy can be useful, especially when combined with visual analog scales [8]. In athletes, it is crucial to know the frequency and the intensity of training. Errors in training technique should be identified. A common training error that is associated with tendinopathy is an abrupt change in the exposure to a given activity; such transition risk may represent an exhaustion of soft tissue cellular adaptation or a mechanical failure response to the rapid increase of load that affects matrix integrity [9]. Finally, the clinician should ask about previous treatment.

Mild Achilles tendinopathy presents as pain 2 cm to 6 cm proximal to the tendon insertion after exercise. As the condition progresses, pain may occur during exercise, and, in severe cases, the pain interferes with activities of daily living [10]. There is good correlation between the severity of the disease and the degree of morning stiffness [10]. Runners classically report pain at the beginning and at the end of their training session, with a pain-free period in the central part of their training session [11].

On clinical examination, both lower limbs should be exposed in their entirety, and the patient should be examined standing and prone. The foot and the heel should be inspected for any malalignment, deformity, obvious asymmetry in the tendon size, localized thickening, Haglund heel, and any previous scars. The Achilles tendon should be palpated for tenderness, increased local temperature, thickening, nodules, and crepitation [12]. The tendon's excursion is estimated to determine any tightness. The "painful arc" sign helps to distinguish between tendon and paratenon lesions. In paratendinopathy, the area of maximum thickening and tenderness remains fixed in relation to the malleoli from full dorsi- to plantarflexion, whereas lesions within the tendon move with ankle

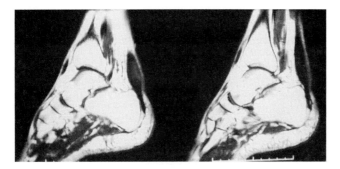

Fig. 1. MRI images demonstrating diffuse fusiform enlargement of the tendon consistent with Achilles tendinopathy. The lack of peritendinous edema suggests isolated tendinopathy of the main body of the Achilles tendon with no paratenon involvement.

motion [13]. There often is a discrete nodule, whose tenderness decreases markedly or disappears when the tendon is put under tension [7,14].

Imaging

The readers are referred to the article by Bleakney and White (elsewhere in this issue) for an exhaustive discussion on this topic. Briefly, we use MRI to evaluate the various stages of chronic degeneration and differentiation between paratendinopathy and tendinopathy of the main body of the tendon (Fig. 1). Because of the high sensitivity of MRI, the data should be interpreted with caution and correlated to the patient's symptoms [4]. Although ultrasonography is operator-dependent, it correlates well with histopathologic finding [15]; we use it as a primary imaging method (Fig. 2). Thickening of the Achilles tendon is detected easily with both methods. If despite ultrasonography the situation

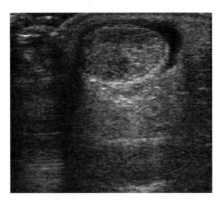

Fig. 2. Ultrasonagraphic findings of Achilles tendinopathy.

remains unclear, an additional MRI study should be performed and, together with the clinical diagnosis, indications for surgery can be made more efficiently [16]. One of the main advantages of ultrasonography over other imaging modalities is its interactive facility, by virtue of its ability to concentrate on the symptomatic area with the use of transducers [17]. Ultrasonography and MRI imaging have a high incidence of false positive findings [4,18].

Management

Management of Achilles tendinopathy is more an art than a science [19]. Few randomized, prospective, placebo-controlled trials exist to assist in choosing the best evidence-based treatment. The current management regimens for chronic Achilles tendinopathy vary significantly, and many are based on little sound scientific support [20–22]. There is a lack of prospective studies evaluating their effectiveness in the management of the disorder, the limited knowledge of the natural history of the condition, the lack of comparative trials, and the majority of the current management strategies based on retrospective scientific support or empirical evidence alone.

Nonoperative management

The conservative care of chronic Achilles tendinopathy encompasses a variety of management strategies, with little scientific basis. Recent prospective studies have led to some success with alternative nonoperative techniques.

Traditional nonoperative management protocols are based on symptom modification strategies [21]. This includes the use of activity-modification strategies, rest, inflammation control therapies, correction of training errors, correction of limb malalignment, flexibility enhancement, muscle strengthening techniques, equipment use modifications, physical therapy regimens and modalities (eg, heat, ultrasound, electrical stimulation), short-term immobilization, and other traditional conservative measures [20–22]. An 8-year observational study showed that traditional nonoperative management was unsuccessful in 29% of 83 patients who had acute or subchronic Achilles tendinopathy [44]. Other studies described a 35% to 50% failure rate with nonsurgical management [23,24].

Anti-inflammatory therapies

Traditionally, nonsteroidal anti-inflammatory drugs have been used in the early phase of Achilles tendinopathy, and are prescribed occasionally for chronic Achilles tendinopathy. Recent scientific evidence does not support the use of such drugs because no chemical markers of inflammation have been associated with the disorder, particularly in the chronic stage. Biopsy specimens have shown a lack of inflammatory cell infiltration; in vivo studies by Alfredson [25] demonstrated a lack of inflammation in patients who had chronic Achilles tendinopathy. In a double-blinded, placebo-controlled study, piroxicam was of no greater benefit than placebo in the management of chronic Achilles tendinopathy [26]. Finally, recent evidence suggests that, paradoxically, the use of nonsteroidal anti-inflammatory drugs for the treatment of tendon inflammation might increase the levels of leukotriene B(4) within the tendon and potentially contribute to the development of tendinopathy [27]. In our practice, we do not recommend oral anti-inflammatories in the management of overuse Achilles tendinopathy; however, they still have a role in tendinopathy that is secondary to inflammatory arthritides.

The role of systemic or local corticosteroids in the management of Achilles tendinopathy also is debated widely [22,28–31]. Peritendinous injections of corticosteroids have been associated with spontaneous rupture of the Achilles tendon. In a recent retrospective study that examined the safety of fluoroscopically-guided low-volume peritendinous corticosteroid injection for Achilles tendinopathy, however, no major complications and only one minor complication (skin discoloration) were reported [32].

A meta-analysis of the complications that were associated with cortisone in the management of Achilles tendinopathy [22] concluded that insufficient data exist to determine accurately the risk of rupture with this drug; similar conclusions were reached in a more recent systematic review [2]. The efficacy of cortisone injections in the management of the disorder also is defined poorly; some series suggested a 40% improvement [32], whereas others suggested no improvement when compared with placebo [31]. In our experience, if the patient presents in the early phase of the condition, and the injection is administered using short-acting corticosteroids in the peritendinous space, this management option is associated with minimal complications [2,29,32]. Intratendinous injections of steroid in animal studies showed reduction in tendon strength with a potential risk of rupture for several weeks following injection (Fig. 3) [33]. A recent article showed that intratendinous injections of corticosteroids can be used in the early phases of the condition; however, these investigators reported on only five patients [34], one of whom relapsed after 199 days. We do not recommend intratendinous injections.

Several other drugs, such as low-dose heparin, glycosaminoglycan, and aprotinin, have been used in the management of peri- and intratendinous pathology [21,35,36]. One of us (NM) routinely uses aprotinin in the management of Achilles tendinopathy, with no reported adverse effects over the course of the last 15 years [35].

Sclerosing agents

Recently, patients who had Achilles tendinopathy were managed with ultrasound-guided injection of a sclerosing agent (polidocanol) to decrease the

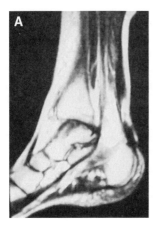
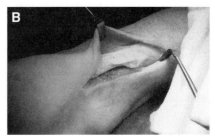

Fig. 3. 28-year-old world ranked squash player who had received three previous corticosteroid injections with an acute exacerbation of pain with long-standing tendinopathy. MRI (*A*) and intraoperative findings (*B*) reveal a partial tear of the Achilles tendon.

neovascularization that was detected in chronic midportion Achilles tendinosis [21,37–39]. Ultrasound and color Doppler studies have demonstrated the presence of neovascularization outside and inside the ventral tendon in areas of tendinopathy [21,39]. The investigators hypothesized that this neovascularization and the nerve fibers that are associated with these neovessels mediate the pain that is associated with Achilles tendinopathy. Hence, by ablation of these neovessels, the underlying pathophysiologic condition is remedied with improvement in discomfort [21,39]. Sclerosing management has given good short-term results in a small series of patients [21]. For an excellent review on this topic, the reader is referred to the article by Alfredson elsewhere in this issue.

Physical therapy modalities

Physical therapy has been used extensively. Specific therapy protocols have focused on concentric strengthening, eccentric strengthening, stretching based protocols, and other management regimens with accompanying modalities. Of all of the modalities, heavy-load eccentric calf muscle training program was the only one tested in a scientific manner, with great efficacy in multiple studies [25,40–42]. Eccentric training is superior to concentric training in decreasing pain in chronic Achilles tendinopathy [41,42]; 81% to 89% of patients report resolution of symptoms. The mechanism by which improvement occurs may be due to an alteration of the tendon's inherent tensile properties or by lengthening of the muscle–tendon unit with stretch. For an excellent review on this topic, the reader is referred to the article by Alfredson elsewhere in this issue.

Vasodilatation techniques

In animal models, topical nitric oxide is effective for the management of fractures and cutaneous wounds through mechanisms that may include stimulation of collagen synthesis in fibroblasts. A recent prospective, randomized, double-blind, placebo-controlled trial that involved 65 patients (84 Achilles tendons) compared continuous application of topical glyceryl trinitrate with rehabilitation alone for the management of noninsertional Achilles tendinopathy. The group that used topical glyceryl trinitrate experienced reduced pain and improved outcomes; 78% of tendons in this group were asymptomatic with activities of daily living at 6 months, compared with 49% of tendons in the group that received placebo [43].

Nonoperative results

Of 83 patients who had acute or subacute Achilles tendinopathy who were followed up for 8 years [44], all were managed nonoperatively initially. At 8 years, 94% of patients were asymptomatic or had only mild pain with exercise, and 84% were able to return to full activity and recreation; however, 29% of the 83 patients failed to improve with conservative management and required surgery. These findings are consistent with previous studies that suggested an approximate 25% failure rate of nonoperative management. Decreased success of conservative management is associated with increased age, prolonged duration of symptoms, and the occurrence of tendinopathic changes. Forty-one percent of the 83 patients in that study developed overuse symptoms of the contralateral Achilles tendon over the follow-up period. Patients may show intratendinous changes in the asymptomatic contralateral tendon at ultrasonography or MRI, but only unilateral symptoms. Both scenarios highlight the lack of understanding of the nociceptive pain-generating mechanisms that are associated with the disorder.

Operative management

Surgery is indicated for patients in whom nonoperative management has failed. The appropriate timing of surgery is controversial, although generally, failure to return the patient's desired level of activities after 3 to 6 months of conservative management justifies surgical intervention. Surgical intervention in chronic Achilles tendinopathy has a success rate of 75% to 100% [2,5,10,15, 45–57]; however, many of these outcome studies have limited validity because of significant methodologic limitations [58]. Some of the difficulties in interpreting the efficacy of surgical intervention in the management of Achilles tendinopathy include the undefined natural history of the disease process, the retrospective nature of many of these investigations, minimal inclusion of objective result evaluations, the lack of comparative operative versus nonoperative trials, and the common inclusion of many coexisting Achilles tendon disorders without strict inclusion criteria. Improved postsurgical status may be related to the natural history of the disorder, extended postoperative immobilization, or the extensive postoperative rehabilitation program.

When surgery is undertaken, the surgeon is spoilt for choice. Clinical examination is critical in guiding the appropriate procedure; if clinical examination is not fully rewarding, diagnostic imaging studies may be necessary to guide surgical planning.

Open exploration and debridement

The most widely used procedure involves a straight longitudinal incision that is placed medially [59] or laterally [30] to expose the diseased tendon. Both approaches yield excellent results. We prefer the medial approach because it avoids the sural nerve and allows for easy access to the flexor hallucis longus if augmentation is necessary (see later discussion). One of us (NM) prefers to use the tendon of peroneus brevis; the peroneal compartment of the leg can be accessed easily, even through a medial skin approach (Fig. 4) [47]. After division of the crural fascia, the paratenon is incised longitudinally, and macroscopic areas of tendinopathy are approached by way of elliptical excision of the diseased superficial portion of the tendon. The area of intrasubstance tendinopathy is debrided extensively. The thickened area of abnormal tendon is obvious and palpable pre- and intraoperatively. In tendons with central core degeneration or in instances where obvious disease is not present, diagnostic imaging allows precise identification of the area of tendon pathology. These areas can be approached at surgery by way of vertical incisions over the relevant portion of the tendon. At times, although the tendon may be thickened, MRI or ultrasound imaging does not demonstrate any discrete signal changes within the tendon. In these cases, we still perform up to three longitudinal tenotomies, given the beneficial effect of such procedure on tendon healing and vascularization [16,18]. Side-to-side suture or a turn-down tendon flap are used in North America to reinforce the tendon if extensive debridement has been performed [15,56,57], but they are not popular in Europe [47].

The underlying mechanism of tendon healing and repair with surgical intervention is poorly understood. Ordered revascularization of the tendon occurs during healing as well; therefore, we recommend avoiding posterior dissection to maintain blood supply to the tendon.

Augmentation/reconstruction

After a thorough debridement of the diseased tendon tissue, occasionally the remaining tendon is of insufficient substance for primary repair. Because of the bulbous nature of the diseased tendon, even after an extensive debridement, sufficient tissue often exists for adequate side-to-side suture reapproximation

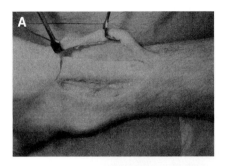
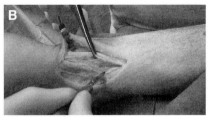
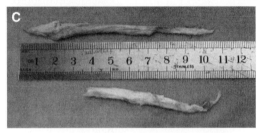
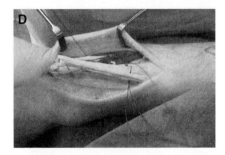
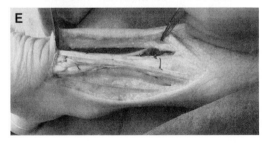

Fig. 4. (A) 22-year-old international rugby player who had widespread Achilles tendinopathy and had received corticosteroid injection treatments with intraoperative widespread tendinosis that was treated with longitudinal tenotomy. (B) Vast degeneration extends through essentially the entire tendon. After extensive excision of diseased tendon (C), reconstruction was performed with a peroneus brevis tendon transfer (D, E). The patient was able to return to rugby 7 months following the procedure.

with minimal compromise. Although the threshold of tendon excision after which augmentation is biologically and biomechanically necessary is not defined clearly, if less than 50% of tendon debridement is required we do not perform an augmentation. If more than 50% of the tendon is debrided, augmentation may be necessary [59]. Options include turn-down patches or flaps for smaller defects, or autogenous tendon transfer augmentation procedures for larger defects (ie, flexor hallucis longus, peroneal brevis, flexor digitorum longus). Recently, the use of flexor hallucis longus (FHL) transfer for the management of defects of the Achilles that require augmentation after debridement produced excellent results, and can be performed safely from a single posteromedial approach with minimal morbidity (Fig. 5) [60]. If a large defect requires greater tendon length or substance for reinforcement, this is accomplished by way of a second midfoot incision [61]. When performing this procedure for Achilles tendinopathy, this additional length usually is not necessary, and occasionally, can be a hindrance when attempting to obtain firm fixation. We secure the transferred flexor hallucis longus tendon to the calcaneus with a biointerference screw; this additional tendon length may prevent placing proper tension because the graft is unable to be passed easily through the os calcis. Additionally, in this scenario, if the tendon is looped back on itself or to the remaining Achilles tendon, this may become excessively large. This transfer allows excellent vascular supply given the large FHL muscle belly close to the tendinopathic Achilles tendon. This technique should be used with caution in elite athletes and runners, especially if involved in American and Australian football, rugby, or soccer. Normally, FHL harvest produces minimal morbidity; however, in these patients, the slight loss of hallux flexion strength may have a significant detrimental impact on performance.

We have recently used Achilles bone–tendon allografts for the management of significant defects of the Achilles. Occasionally, this has been necessary after a planned primary extensive debridement, but more often has been used as an excellent option for management after a failed previous reconstructive/augmentation procedure in a patient who had a significant defect. An extensile approach that extends distally over the midline of the os calcis is the preferred procedure. The patient's Achilles tendon is debrided thoroughly to excise all remaining degenerative tendon tissue. A trough is created in the posterior calcaneus, and the entire remaining Achilles attachment is detached with the 3-mm to 4-mm bone trough resection of the posterior os calcis. The calcaneal portion of the bone–tendon allograft is beveled correspondingly, and a similar 3-mm to 4-mm wedge with the Achilles tendon insertion is secured to the native os calcis and secured with internal fixation. The proximal allograft tendon is secured to the patient's native Achilles tendon with the foot in maximal plantarflexion. The construct is tensioned maximally and repaired in this overtensioned position.

The pain relief that is associated with Achilles allograft reconstruction probably is related to the debridement of the associated neurogenic nociceptive stimulators within the diseased tissue. The advantage of the allograft is the reliable distal bone-to-bone healing. The proximal allograft to native Achilles healing occurred reliably in our experience as well, although slight laxity in the

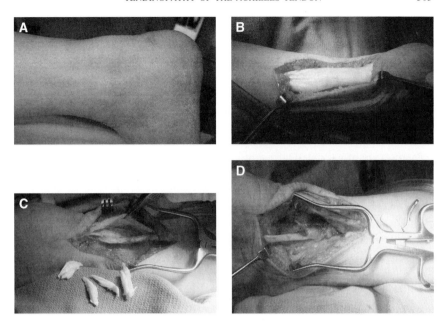

Fig. 5. Clinical (*A*) and intraoperative findings (*B*) of a patient who had extensive tendinopathy of the main body of the Achilles tendon. After extensive debridement (*C*), reconstruction is performed with flexor hallucis longus tendon harvested through a posterior approach (*D*).

repair may occur with incorporation at this level; this is our rationale for initial overtensioning of the repair.

Percutaneous technique

In patients who have isolated Achilles tendinopathy with no peritendinous involvement and a well-defined nodular lesion that is less than 2.5 cm long, we have used multiple percutaneous longitudinal tenotomies [46,47,62]. An ultrasonographic scan can be used to confirm the precise location of the area of tendinopathy. If the multiple percutaneous tenotomies are performed in the absence of paratendinopathy, the outcome is comparable to that of open procedures. In addition, the technique is simple, and can be performed in an outpatient setting under local anesthesia without a tourniquet. Attention to detail is necessary, because complications are possible, even in minimally invasive procedures.

This technique, with or without the use of ultrasound guidance, may produce approximately 75% success if patients who have concomitant paratendinopathy are excluded [62]. Although the rationale for the improvement is not clear, experimental evidence suggests that intratendinous neoangiogenesis occurs, with a return to normal biochemistry of tendon which is beneficial to healing [16,18,62].

Postoperative rehabilitation

Rehabilitation protocols after Achilles reconstruction are varied; even among institutions the specific program that is used is "individualized," based on the degree of degenerative changes or the procedure performed. Generally, postoperative immobilization is standard with all protocols, with the duration of immobilization lasting from 2 to 8 weeks in most series. The position of immobilization is variable, with some recommendations of neutral position, plantarflexion of varying degrees, or to a point where gentle tension is placed on the tendon. We use 2 weeks of immobilization in a weight-bearing, below knee synthetic cast, with range-of-motion exercises after that time with concomitant stretching. Progressive strengthening and motion rehabilitation in a supervised program is then recommended. In a prospective evaluation of supervised stepwise flexibility and strength training (concentric and eccentric) during the first year after reconstruction for Achilles tendinopathy, the injured extremity was significantly weaker than the nonoperated side for 6 to 12 months [1]. No improvement in time to strength recovery was noted by decreasing the initial immobilization. Most investigators recommend a gradual return to sports when strength has been regained [1]; however, this definition often is vague, and no criteria explicitly guide return to sports. Saltzman et al recommended return to play for competitive sports at 5 to 6 months after injury (67). Alfredson et al [25] prospectively evaluated the degree of calcaneal bone loss postoperatively. They demonstrated that when patients were allowed to return to sports (at ~6 to 12 months), the calcaneus still had a significantly lower bone mass than the contralateral side; this suggests vulnerability with early return to competitive activities. Although we allow patients to return to activity as early as possible with pain as the guide of limitation, we caution patients that postoperative recovery and rehabilitation from these procedures can be extensive and can continue for up to 1 year after surgical correction.

In our series of patients who had bone–tendon allograft reconstruction for massive Achilles defects, we used a conservative rehabilitation regime. Patients were immobilized in a cast in plantarflexion (~20–25°) with slight tension placed on the reconstruction and gastro–soleus complex for approximately 2 weeks, which gradually progressed toward neutral by 6 weeks. At 6 weeks, patients began rehabilitation and a weight-bearing program with a focus on eccentric training.

Surgical results

Open debridement procedures have yielded good to excellent results in 75% to 100% of patients [2,5,10,15,45–57]. Other investigators have, however, reported significantly worse results. Maffulli et al [53] reported on 14 athletes at 35 months who had chronic recalcitrant Achilles tendinopathy with an evident lesion of the main body of the Achilles tendon that was managed with open exploration and debridement. Only 5 of 14 patients experienced an excellent or good result, despite a subsequent procedure in 6 of 14 patients. The same investigators reported good to excellent results in 77% of patients at 1.5 to 11 years of follow-up after percutaneous longitudinal tenotomy [62]. This led to an increased interest in this procedure, which we also have used with good results.

Our early results with bone–tendon os calcis Achilles allograft have been encouraging. In all patients, the allograft is functional at early follow-up; patients demonstrate excellent plantarflexion strength and push-off. Nevertheless, the gastro-soleus complex, when tested using isokinetic dynamometry, is weaker than the contralateral.

Complications that are associated with surgical management are not rare [44], and in most series, mainly involve wound-healing complications. Paavola et al [56] studied the complication rates that were associated with chronic Achilles tendon overuse injuries. Forty-six of 432 patients (11%) developed some complication, most commonly skin edge necrosis (14 cases) or superficial wound infections (11 cases). Other complications included seroma or hematoma formation (10 cases), fibrotic reactions or scar formations (5 cases), sural neuritis (4 cases), new partial rupture (1 case), or thrombosis (1 case). Fourteen patients required reoperation. Although excellent results often are reported with surgery, approximately 20% of patients may require reoperation and approximately 3% to 5% give up their athletic career because of therapy-resistant pain in the Achilles tendon [40].

Summary

Recent research has improved our understanding of the pathophysiology of Achilles tendinopathy. Chemical inflammation is not a feature of chronic overuse Achilles tendinopathy, and neovascularization in the peritendinous areas or a possible "neurogenic inflammation" that is caused by irritation of mechanoreceptors or triggering of nociceptive receptors may exist. Emerging nonoperative management and heavy-load eccentric strengthening protocols that are based on these theories have yielded encouraging early results. Nevertheless, significant lapses in our knowledge remain. Traditionally, operative management has produced good to excellent results; however, randomized, controlled studies that compare different surgical procedures and prospective evaluation of patient outcomes are necessary to establish the true efficacy of these procedures.

References

[1] Jozsa LG, Kannus P. Human tendons: anatomy, physiology, and pathology. Champaign (IL): Human Kinetics; 1997.

[2] Maffulli N, Kader D. Tendinopathy of tendo achillis. J Bone Joint Surg Br 2002;84:1–8.

[3] el Hawary R, Stanish WD, Curwin SL. Rehabilitation of tendon injuries in sport. Sports Med 1997;24:347–58.

[4] Leadbetter WB. Cell-matrix response in tendon injury. Clin Sports Med 1992;11(3):533–78.

[5] Astrom M. Partial rupture in chronic Achilles tendinopathy. A retrospective analysis of 342 cases. Acta Orthop Scand 1998;69(4):404–7.

[6] Benazzo F, Maffulli N. An operative approach to Achilles tendinopathy. Sports Med Arthroscopy Rev 2000;8:96–101.

[7] Kvist M. Achilles tendon overuse injuries [master's thesis]. Oulu (Finland): University of Oulu; 1991.

[8] Sports-induced inflammation. Clinical and basic science concepts (symposium series). Parkridge: American Academy of Orthopaedic Surgeons; 1990.

[9] Leadbetter W. Soft tissue athletic injury in sports injuries: mechanisms prevention and treatment. Baltimore (MD): Williams & Wilkins; 1994.

[10] Binfield PM, Maffulli N. Surgical management of common tendinopathies of the lower limb. Sports Exerc Injury 1997;3:116–22.

[11] Rogers BS, Leach RE. Achilles tendinitis. Foot Ankle Clin 1996;1(2):249–59.

[12] Teitz CC, Garrett WEJ, Miniaci A, et al. Tendon problems in athletic individuals. Instr Course Lect 1997;46:569–82.

[13] Williams JG. Achilles tendon lesions in sport. Sports Med 1986;3(2):114–35.

[14] Maffulli N, Kenward MG, Testa V, et al. The clinical diagnosis of Achilles tendinopathy. Clin J Sport Med 2003;13:11–5.

[15] Rolf C, Movin T. Etiology, histopathology, and outcome of surgery in achillodynia. Foot Ankle Int 1997;18(9):565–9.

[16] Neuhold A, Stiskal M, Kainberger F, et al. Degenerative Achilles tendon disease: assessment by magnetic resonance and ultrasonography. Eur J Radiol 1992;14(3):213–20.

[17] Gibbon WW. Musculoskeletal ultrasound. Baillieres Clin Rheumatol 1996;10(4):561–88.

[18] Merk H. High-resolution real-time sonography in the diagnosis of Achilles tendon diseases. Ultraschall Med 1989;10(4):192–7.

[19] Khan KM, Maffulli N. Tendinopathy: an Achilles' heel for athletes and clinicians. Clin J Sport Med 1998;8(3):151–4.

[20] Kellett J. Acute soft tissue injuries—a review of the literature. Med Sci Sports Exerc 1986;18(5):489–500.

[21] Öhberg L, Alfredson H. Ultrasound guided sclerosis of neovessels in painful chronic Achilles tendinosis: pilot study of a new treatment. Br J Sports Med 2002;36:173–7.

[22] Speed CA. Corticosteroid injections in tendon lesions. BMJ 2001;323(7309):382–6.

[23] Maffulli N, Khan KM, Puddu G. Overuse tendon conditions: time to change a confusing terminology. Arthroscopy 1998;14(8):840–3.

[24] Saltzman CL, Tearse DS. Achilles tendon injuries. J Am Acad Orthop Surg 1998;6:316–25.

[25] Alfredson H. Chronic midportion Achilles tendinopathy: an update on research and treatment. Clin Sports Med 2003;22:10–3.

[26] Astrom M, Westlin N. No effect of piroxicam on Achilles tendinopathy. A randomized study of 70 patients. Acta Orthop Scand 1992;63:631–4.

[27] Li Z, Yang G, Khan M, Stone D, et al. Inflammatory response of human tendon fibroblasts to cyclic mechanical stretching. Am J Sports Med 2004;32(2):435–40.

[28] Capasso G, Testa V, Maffulli N, et al. Aprotinin, corticosteroids and normosaline in the management of patellar tendinopathy in athletes: a prospective randomized study. Sports Exercise and Injury 1997;3:111–5.

[29] Fredberg U. Local corticosteroid injection in sport: review of literature and guidelines for treatment. Scand J Med Sci Sports 1997;7:131–9.

[30] Shrier I, Matheson GO, Kohl III HW. Achilles tendonitis: are corticosteroid injections useful or harmful? Clin J Sport Med 1996;6:245–50.

[31] Speed CA. Fortnightly review: Corticosteroid injections in tendon lesions. BMJ 2001;323: 382–6.

[32] Gill S, Gebke M, Mattson S, et al. Fluoroscopically guided low-volume peritendinous corticosteroid injection for Achilles tendinopathy: a safety study. J Bone Joint Surg 2004;86: 802–6.

[33] Hugate R, Pennypacker J, Saunders M, et al. The effects of intratendinous and retrocalcaneal intrabursal injections of corticosteroid on the biomechanical properties of rabbit Achilles tendons. J Bone Joint Surg Am 2004;86-A(4):794–801.

[34] Clancy WGJ, Neidhart D, Brand RL. Achilles tendonitis in runners: a report of five cases. Am J Sports Med 1976;4(2):46–57.

[35] Capasso G, Maffulli N, Testa V, et al. Preliminary results with peritendinous protease inhibitor injections in the management of Achilles tendinitis. J Sports Traumatol Rel Res 1993;15:37–43.

[36] Owoeye I, Spielholz NI, Fetto J, et al. Low-intensity pulsed galvanic current and the healing of tenotomized rat Achilles tendons: preliminary report using load-to-breaking measurements. Arch Phys Med Rehabil 1987;68(7):415–8.

[37] Jackson BA, Schwane JA, Starcher BC. Effect of ultrasound therapy on the repair of Achilles tendon injuries in rats. Med Sci Sports Exerc 1991;23(2):171–6.

[38] Koenig MJ, Torp-Pedersen S, Qvistgaard E, et al. Preliminary results of colour Doppler-guided intratendinous glucocorticoid injection for Achilles tendinitis in five patients. Scand J Med Sci Sports 2004;14(2):100–6.

[39] Öhberg L, Lorentzon R, Alfredson H. Neovascularisation in Achilles tendons with painful tendinosis but not in normal tendons: an ultrasonographic investigation. Knee Surg Sports Traumatol Arthrosc 2001;9:233–8.

[40] Alfredson H, Lorentzon R. Chronic Achilles tendinosis: recommendations for treatment and prevention. Sports Med 2000;29:135–46.

[41] Alfredson H, Pietilä T, Jonsson P, et al. Heavy-load eccentric calf muscle training for the treatment of chronic Achilles tendinosis. Am J Sports Med 1998;26:360–6.

[42] Silbernagel KG, Thomee R, Thomee P, et al. Eccentric overload training for patients with chronic Achilles tendon pain-a randomised controlled study with reliability testing of the evaluation methods. Scand J Med Sci Sports 2001;11:197–206.

[43] Paoloni J, Appleyard R, Nelson J, et al. Topical glycerol trinitrate treatment of chronic noninsertional Achilles tendinopathy: a randomized, double-blind, placebo-controlled trial. J Bone Joint Surg 2004;86-A(5):916–22.

[44] Paavola M, Kannus P, Paakkala T, et al. Long-term prognosis of patients with Achilles tendinopathy. An observational 8-year follow-up study. Am J Sports Med 2000;28:634–42.

[45] Almekinders LC, Temple JD. Etiology, diagnosis, and treatment of tendonitis: an analysis of the literature. Med Sci Sports Exerc 1998;30:1183–90.

[46] Angermann P, Hovgaard D. Chronic Achilles tendinopathy in athletic individuals: results of conservative and surgical treatments. Foot Ankle Int 1999;20:304–6.

[47] Clement DB, Taunton JE, Smart GW. Achilles tendinitis and peritendinitis: etiology and treatment. Am J Sports Med 1984;12(3):179–84.

[48] Johnston E, Scranton P, Pfeffer GB. Chronic disorders of the Achilles tendon: results of conservative and surgical treatments. Foot Ankle Int 1997;18:570–4.

[49] Kvist M. Achilles tendon injuries in athletes. Sports Med 1994;18:173–201.

[50] Lehto MU, Järvinen M, Suominen P. Chronic Achilles peritendinitis and retrocalcanear bursitis. Long-term follow-up of surgically treated cases. Knee Surg Sports Traumatol Arthrosc 1994; 2:182–5.

[51] Leppilahti J, Karpakka J, Gorra A, et al. Surgical treatment of overuse injuries to the Achilles tendon. Clin J Sport Med 1994;4:100–7.

[52] Saltzman CL, Tearse DS. Achilles tendon injuries. J Am Acad Orthop Surg 1998;6:316–25.

[53] Maffulli N, Binfield PM, Moore D, et al. Surgical decompression of chronic central core lesions of the Achilles tendon. Am J Sports Med 1999;27(6):747–52.

[54] Morberg P, Jerre R, Sward L, et al. Long-term results after surgical management of partial Achilles tendon ruptures. Scand J Med Sci Sports 1997;7:299–303.

[55] Paavola M, Kannus P, Orava S, et al. Surgical treatment for chronic Achilles tendinopathy: a prospective 7-month follow-up study. Br J Sports Med 2002;36:178–82.

[56] Paavola M, Orava S, Leppilahti J, et al. Chronic Achilles tendon overuse injury: complications after surgical treatment. Am J Sports Med 2000;28:77–82.

[57] Sandmeier R, Renström PA. Diagnosis and treatment of chronic tendon disorders in sports. Scand J Med Sci Sports 1997;7:96–106.

[58] Tallon C, Coleman BD, Khan KM, et al. Outcome of surgery for chronic Achilles tendinopathy. A critical review. Am J Sports Med 2001;29:315–20.

[59] Schepsis AA, Leach RE. Surgical management of Achilles tendinitis. Am J Sports Med 1987; 15:308–15.

[60] Den Hartog BD. Flexor hallucis longus transfer for chronic Achilles tendonosis. Foot Ankle Int 2003;24(3):233–7.

[61] Tashjian RZ, Hur J, Sullivan RJ, et al. Flexor hallucis longus transfer for repair of chronic Achilles tendinopathy. Foot Ankle Int 2003;24(9):673–6.

[62] Testa V, Giovanni C, Benazzo F, et al. Management of Achilles tendinopathy by ultrasound-guided percutaneous tenotomy. Med Sci Sports Exerc 2002;34:573–80.

ELSEVIER
SAUNDERS

Foot Ankle Clin N Am
10 (2005) 309–320

FOOT AND
ANKLE CLINICS

Insertional Achilles Tendinopathy

Murali Krishna Sayana, MBBS, MS, AFRCSI, Nicola Maffulli, MD, MS, PhD, FRCS(Orth)*

Department of Trauma and Orthopaedics, University Hospital of North Staffordshire, Keele University School of Medicine, Thornburrow Drive, Stoke-on-Trent, ST4 7QB, UK

Achilles tendinopathy is one of the conditions that causes posterior heel pain. Clain and Baxter [1] introduced the terms insertional and noninsertional Achilles tendinopathy with a view to plan management better. Insertional tendinopathy had a prevalence of 20% in a surgical and histopathologic survey of 163 patients who had chronic Achilles tendinopathy [2]. In a consecutive series of 432 patients who had chronic Achilles overuse injury in Finland, 107 (24.7%) had insertional Achilles pathology. Of these, 5% (21 patients) had pure insertional tendinopathy, and 20% (86 patients) had calcaneal bursitis alone or in combination with insertional tendinopathy [3].

The incidence of Achilles insertional tendinopathy is not well established. It was reported as the most common form of Achilles tendinopathy in athletes who presented to an outpatient clinic [4]. Conversely, 5% to 20% of the Achilles tendinopathy were of the insertional variety [3,5]. Insertional tendinopathy often is diagnosed in older, less athletic, overweight individuals [6], and in older athletes [7].

In this article we specifically concentrate on Achilles insertional tendinopathy. We shall not discuss Haglund's deformity and retrocalcaneal bursitis in detail. We advocate the use of the term "tendinopathy" for a clinical diagnosis that is based on pain, swelling (diffuse or localized), and impaired performance. We use the suffix "osis" or "itis" only after histopathologic examination of the affected tendons has confirmed degeneration or inflammation [8]. Although, insertional tendinopathy of the Achilles tendon is often described as "true inflammation" within the tendon [7], the histology from 22 patients who had

---

* Corresponding author.
E-mail address: n.maffulli@keele.ac.uk (N. Maffulli).

1083-7515/05/$ – see front matter © 2005 Elsevier Inc. All rights reserved.
doi:10.1016/j.fcl.2005.01.010
foot.theclinics.com

recalcitrant calcific insertional Achilles tendinopathy showed fibrocartilaginous or calcifying degeneration close to the area of calcific tendinopathy. There was disorganization of the tendon substance with no evidence of intratendinous inflammatory reaction [9]. We advocate the use of the term "Achilles insertional tendinopathy" in this context.

Anatomy

The gastrocnemius muscle merges with the soleus to form the Achilles tendon. It has a round upper part, and is mostly flat in its distal 4 cm. Its fibers spiral through 90° and increase the release of stored energy during locomotion [10]. The Achilles tendon inserts into the posterior surface of the calcaneus, which can be divided into three areas [11]:

- A triangular bursal area with superior apex. The tendon is not inserted in this area.
- A rough quadrilateral area inferior to the bursal area that provides insertion to the central part of the Achilles tendon.
- A triangular inferior area with inferior apex. This gives attachment to fascial structures that are continuous with the plantar fascia below and with the sheath of the Achilles tendon above.

The insertion of the Achilles tendon, the posterior aspect of the calcaneus, the retrocalcaneal bursa, and the pretendinous bursa constitute the posterior aspect of the heel. The enthesis, the bursa, and the bursal walls form a complex insertional region that protects the Achilles tendon and the posterior aspect of the heel.

Histology

The osteo-tendinous junction of the Achilles consists of tendon, fibrocartilage, and bone. Milz et al [12] used the distribution of type II collagen in sagittal sections of the Achilles tendon to reconstruct the three-dimensional (3-D) shape and position of three fibrocartilages (sesamoid, periosteal, and enthesis) that are associated with its insertion. A close correspondence between the shape and position of the sesamoid and periosteal fibrocartilages was found. The former protects the tendon from compression during dorsiflexion of the foot, and the latter protects the superior tuberosity of the calcaneus. The 3-D reconstructions that used the zone of calcified enthesis, fibrocartilage, and the subchondral bone showed complex interlocking between calcified fibrocartilage and bone at the insertion site; this is of fundamental importance in anchoring the tendon to the bone.

Merkel et al [13] studied 11 insertional tendinopathy (including two Achilles tendons) specimens using light and electronic microscopy, and enzyme histochemistry. The pathologic changes of insertional tendinopathy consisted of edema, mucoid degeneration, disruption of collagen bundles, necroses, small hemorrhages, and calcification. Acid mucopolysaccharides may be present in lakelike accumulations between collagen fibers, in contrast to neutral collagens that are seen in aging. Small bony particles lay within the cartilaginous portion of the insertion. Also, there were areas with proliferating blood vessels within tendon tissue with lymphocytes and histiocytes that suggested a reparative process. There was increased activity of NADP-diaphorase, lactate dehydrogenase (LDH) in these tendon samples. β-glucuronidase and alkaline phosphatase enzymes were also found in these samples, though their activity was lower compared to NADP-diaphorase, LDH. Electron microscopy showed marked submicroscopic calcification and fibrillar degeneration.

Etiopathophysiology

Classically, overuse and poor training habits are considered to be the main etiology of Achilles insertional tendinopathy. Spur formation and calcification at the Achilles insertion is attributed to gradual repetitive traction force. Benjamin et al [14] studied enthesophyte formation in rats compared with human specimens. Bony spurs can develop in the Achilles tendon without the need for preceding microtears or inflammatory reactions, and form by endochondral ossification of enthesis fibrocartilage. The increased surface area that is created at the tendon–bone junction may be an adaptive mechanism to ensure the integrity of the interface in response to increased mechanical loads [14].

Tight Achilles tendon, hyperpronation, pes cavus, and obesity can predispose to degeneration, attrition, mechanical abrasion, and chemical irritation that could lead to a chronic inflammatory response at the heel [6].

Lyman et al [15] studied the in vitro strain behavior of the anterior portion of the Achilles tendon as it is affected by the insertional tendinopathy. Relative strain shielding was noticed in this portion of the tendon; this suggests that the role of repetitive tensile loads in the causation of Achilles insertional tendinopathy is complex. These findings may explain the variable therapeutic response that followed measures that were aimed at decreasing tensile loads on the tendon.

A different etiology of insertional tendinopathy recently was suggested based on biomechanical studies (C.N. Maganaris, PhD, personal communication, 2004). There is a distinct tendency to develop cartilage-like or atrophic changes on the stress-shielded side of the enthesis as a response to the lack of tensile load [16,17]. Over long periods, this process may induce a primary degenerative lesion in that area of the tendon. Thus, tendinopathy is not always activity-related, and can be correlated with age; this suggests that insertional tendinopathy would result from stress-shielding, rather than overuse injury.

In many ways, the cartilage-like changes in the enthesis can be considered to be a physiologic adaptation to the compressive loads. Even cartilaginous metaplasia, however, may not allow the tendon to maintain its ability to withstand the high tensile loads in that region. In athletes, certain joint positions may place high tensile loads on the enthesis. As the stress-shielding may have led to tensile weakening over time, an injury may occur more easily in this region. In this manner, insertional tendinopathy could be considered to be an overuse injury, but is predisposed by pre-existing weakening of the tendon.

As the joint changes position, strains in one section of the tendon could produce changes in the opposite direction. Internal shear forces and heat could be generated that produce injury to the cellular or matrix components of the tendon [18]. Accumulation of these injuries could lead to the intratendinous degeneration that is seen in tendinopathy.

Clinical features

Achilles insertional tendinopathy is characterized by early morning stiffness, pain that is localized at the insertion of the Achilles tendon that worsens after exercise, climbing stairs, running on hard surfaces, or heel running. The pain may become constant. There may be a history of a recent increase in training, and poor warm-up or stretching habits. Examination reveals tenderness at the Achilles tendon insertion, thickening or nodularity of the insertion, and limited dorsiflexion of the ankle.

Differential diagnosis

Other causes of posterior heel pain should be considered. Achilles insertional tendinopathy is a localized manifestation of systemic conditions, such as gout, hyperlipidemia, sarcoidosis, diffuse idiopathic skeletal hyperostosis, or seronegative spondyloarthropathies. Systemic corticosteroids and oral fluoroquinolones may induce Achilles insertional tendinopathy. Local conditions, such as Haglund's deformity, retrocalcaneal bursitis, os trigonum, posterior impingement, posterior talar process fracture, flexor hallucis longus tendinopathy, peroneal tendinopathy, tibialis posterior tendinopathy, deltoid ligament sprain, and osteochondral lesions of talus should be ruled out.

Investigations

Radiographs may reveal ossification at the insertion of the Achilles tendon or a spur (fishhook osteophyte) on the superior portion of the calcaneum. Morris et al [19] classified the radio-opacities of the Achilles tendon into three types (Table 1).

Table 1
Radio-opacities of the Achilles tendon

Type I lesion	Etiology
Microtrauma	Shoe counter, work-related irritation
Macrotrauma	Insertion rupture, blunt trauma
Tendinopathy	Overuse, bursitis, calcaneus shape
Foot type	Cavus, rear foot varus, plantarflexed 1st metatarsal
Arthropathy	Gout, rheumatoid, Reiter's, ankylosing spondylitis, diffuse idiopathic skeletal hyperostosis
Metabolic	Renal failure, obesity, hyperparathyroidism, hemochromatosis
Infectious	Acute or chronic syphilis
Type II lesion	
Arthropathy	Articular chondrocalcinosis, pseudogout
Metabolic	Vitamin deficiency
Type III lesion	
Trauma	Burn injury, partial/total tendon rupture
Postsurgery	Primary repair, lengthening, recession
Ischemia	Inherent anatomy
Infectious	Chronic osteomyelitis
Systemic/metabolic	Wilson's disease, hemochromatosis
Congenital	Aperiosteal metaplasia, neural arch deficiency
CNS	Tabes dorsalis

Abbreviation: CNS, central nervous system.
Modified from Morris KL, Giacopelli JA, Granoff D. Classification of radiopaque lesions of tendo Achillis. J Foot Surg 1990;29(6):536.

Type I: radio-opacities at the Achilles insertion or superior pole of the calcaneus. The lesion is present within the tendon and is attached partially or completely to the calcaneus. Bony changes to the calcaneus often are seen in type I lesions. Insertional Achilles tendinopathy causes type I abnormality (Fig. 1).

Type II: intratendinous radio-opacities located at the insertion zone, 1 cm to 3 cm proximal to the Achilles insertion and separated from the calcaneal surface.

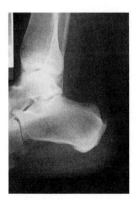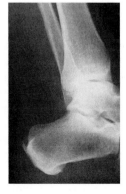

Fig. 1. Bilateral Achilles insertional tendinopathy. Type I.

Table 2
Ultrasonographic classification of insertional Achilles tendon abnormality

Classification	Insertional changes
No alteration	No calcification. Homogeneous fiber structure in the insertional area.
Mild abnormality	Insertional calcification, length 10 mm or less and thickness less than 2 mm. Homogeneous fiber structure in the insertional area.
Moderate abnormality	Insertional calcification, length more than 10 mm and thickness less than 2 mm.
	Slight alterations in the echo structure of tendon in the insertional area.
Severe abnormality	Insertional calcification, length more than 10 mm or thickness more than 2 mm.
	Moderate to severe variety in the echo structure of tendon in the insertional area.

Type III: radio-opacities located proximal to the insertion zone, up to 12 cm above the insertion zone. Type III is subdivided into IIIA (partial tendon calcification) and IIIB (complete tendon calcification).

MRI and ultrasound scan are not needed for diagnosis, but they may help to identify the extent of the intratendinous lesion. An ultrasonographic classification of the Achilles tendon abnormalities that is based on changes at the Achilles tendon insertion was introduced by Paavola et al (Table 2) [20].

Management

Conservative management produces an 85% to 95% success rate [6,21] with rest, ice, modification of training, heel lift, and orthoses. Nonsteroidal anti-inflammatory medications in Achilles tendinopathy may only provide an analgesic effect [22]. Piroxicam showed no benefit over placebo in a randomized controlled trial when it was combined with an initial period of rest followed by stretching and strengthening exercises [23]. Diclofenac reduced the accumulation of inflammatory cells only within the paratenon, but provided no biochemical, mechanical, or functional benefits to the rat Achilles tendon following injury when compared with placebo. Also, no reduction in the accumulation of neutrophils and macrophages was found in the core of the tendon [24].

Modification of training, stretching, and strengthening exercises also are effective; however, eccentric calf muscle training helped only 32% of cases of Achilles insertional tendinopathy compared with 89% of cases of noninsertional tendinopathy [25]. In athletes, nonweight-bearing activities can help to maintain fitness until symptoms improve. Immobilization of the ankle in a below-knee weight-bearing cast or a walker boot can be counterproductive, although it was suggested by some investigators [6,26]. Tendon loading stimulates collagen fiber repair and remodeling. Therefore, complete rest of an injured tendon is not advisable. Ultrasound treatment could be beneficial to control symptoms at the insertion site. We do not use local injections of corticosteroids.

Sclerosing therapy in insertional tendinopathy showed promising results in a pilot study [27]. Polidocanol was injected into local neovessels that were localized by ultrasound and color Doppler. Eight of eleven patients experienced good pain relief, and seven of them had no neovascularization at a mean follow-up of 8 months.

Surgery

Surgery is undertaken if conservative management fails. Various surgical procedures have been described. The principles of surgery include debridement of the calcific or diseased portion of the Achilles insertion, excision of the retrocalcaneal bursa, and resection of the superior prominence. We prefer to reattach the Achilles tendon using bone anchors if one third or more of the insertion is disinserted. Augmentation using tendon transfer is well-described.

Anderson et al [28] studied the surgical management of chronic Achilles tendinopathy in 48 patients that included 27 competitive athletes. Twenty-eight (58%) patients underwent surgery for Achilles insertional tendinopathy with tenolysis, excision of the bursa, or excision of the posterosuperior portion of the calcaneum through a 10-cm medial incision. The recovery in these patients was longer (31 weeks) when compared with an Achilles tenolysis group (22 weeks) with a success rate of 93%.

Calder and Saxby [29] reported their results of intervention in which less than 50% of the tendon was excised (49 heels); the operated ankles were mobilized immediately, free of a cast. There were two failures using this regimen: one patient who had psoriatic arthropathy and another who underwent bilateral simultaneous procedures. Kolodziej et al [30] reported a biomechanical study that concluded that superior-to-inferior resection offers the greatest margin of safety when performing partial resections of the Achilles insertion; as much as 50% of the tendon may be resected safely.

McGarvey et al [31] reported the results on 22 heels that had surgery using a midline-posterior skin incision combined with a central tendon splitting ap-proach for debridement, retrocalcaneal bursectomy, and removal of the cal-caneal bursal projection, as necessary. Twenty of 22 patients were able to return to work or routine activities by 3 months. Only 13 of 22 patients were completely pain-free and were able to return to unlimited activities. Overall, there was an 82% (18 of 22 patients) satisfaction rate with surgery.

Watson et al [32] reported that retrocalcaneal decompression in patients who had insertional Achilles tendinopathy with a calcific spur was less satisfactory when compared with retrocalcaneal decompression in patients who had isolated retrocalcaneal bursitis.

Den Hartog [33] reported the successful use of flexor hallucis longus trans-fer for severe calcific Achilles tendinopathy in 26 patients (29 tendons), in whom conservative treatment had failed and who also had failed tendon debridement or Haglund's resection. These patients were sedentary, overweight, and had chronic symptoms. The American Orthopaedic Foot and Ankle Society ankle-hindfoot scale improved from 41.7 to 90.1. The time to maximum recovery was approximately 6 months. All patients lost flexor strength at the inter-phalangeal joint of the great toe.

Leitze et al [34] recently reported decompression of the retrocalcaneal space using a minimally invasive technique. Patients who had retrocalcaneal bursitis, mechanical impingement, or Achilles insertional tendinopathy who failed to respond to conservative management underwent endoscopic decompression; major calcific insertional tendinopathy of the Achilles tendon was considered to be a contraindication for endoscopic decompression. The advantages of the endoscopic procedure included quicker surgery and fewer complications, al-though the recovery time was similar to open decompression.

We reported on 21 patients who had recalcitrant calcific insertional Achilles tendinopathy who underwent bursectomy, excision of the distal paratenon, disinsertion of the tendon, removal of the calcific deposit, and reinsertion of the Achilles tendon with bone anchors. The outcome of surgical management was rated according to Testa et al [35], using a 4-point functional scale that was validated for the evaluation of long-term results following surgery for ten-dinopathy. Eleven patients reported an excellent result and five reported a good result. The remaining five patients could not return to their normal levels of sporting activity and kept fit by alternative means [9].

Authors' preferred surgical technique

Surgery is performed on a day case basis. Under general anesthesia, the patient is laid prone with a thigh tourniquet that is inflated to 250 mm Hg after the limb has been exsanguinated to provide hemostasis. The Achilles tendon is exposed through a longitudinal incision that is 1 cm medial to the medial border of the tendon, and is extended from the lower one third of the tendon up to 2 cm distal to its calcaneal insertion (Fig. 2). The incision can be extended transversely and laterally in a hockey-stick fashion, if necessary. Sharp dissection is continued to the paratenon, which is dissected from the tendon and excised, taking care to preserve the anterior fat in Kager's triangle and not to injure the mesotenon. The retrocalcaneal bursa is excised, if there is evidence of bursitis. The Achilles tendon is inspected for areas that had lost their normal shining appearance and palpated for areas of softening or thickening. The areas that have lost their normal shining appearance, and the areas that are softer or thicker are explored by way of one to three longitudinal tenotomies; areas of degeneration are excised and sent for histology. The longitudinal tenotomies are not repaired. The area of calcific tendinopathy is identified and its proximal, medial, and lateral edges are defined using the tip of a syringe needle. The calcific area is exposed starting from its proximal and medial aspect. Most patients have at least one third of the Achilles tendon that surrounds the area of

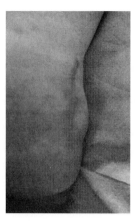

Fig. 2. Well-healed incision on the medial side 6 weeks after surgery. The posterior swelling would take a few months to subside.

calcific tendinopathy detached by sharp dissection; occasionally, a total dis-insertion has to be performed. The area of calcific tendinopathy is excised from the calcaneus. The area of hyaline cartilage at the posterosuperior corner of the calcaneus may be degenerated macroscopically; it is excised using an osteotome and, if needed, its base paired off with bone nibblers. The tendon is reinserted in the calcaneus using bone anchors. Two bone anchors are be used if 33% to 50% of the Achilles tendon is disinserted; three soft bone anchors are used if 50% to 75% of the Achilles tendon is disinserted; four bone anchors are used if 75% or more of the Achilles tendon is disinserted (Fig. 3); and five bone anchors are used if the Achilles tendon is disinserted totally. The Achilles tendon is advanced in a proximal to distal fashion and reinserted in the calca-neum. We normally do not perform a tendon augmentation or a tendon transfer. After release of the tourniquet, hemostasis is achieved by diathermy. The wound is closed in layers using absorbable sutures.

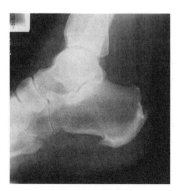
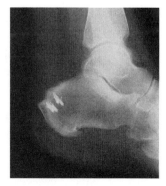

Fig. 3. Four suture anchors in a postoperative radiograph.

Postoperative management

The skin wound is dressed with gauze, and sterile plaster wool is applied. A synthetic below-knee cast, with the ankle plantigrade, is applied. Patients are discharged the day of surgery. Patients are mobilized with crutches under the guidance of a physiotherapist in the immediate postoperative period. Patients are advised to bear weight on the operated leg as tolerated, but are told to keep the leg elevated as much as possible for the first 2 postoperative weeks. The cast is removed 2 weeks after the operation. A synthetic anterior below-knee slab is applied, with the ankle in neutral. The synthetic slab is secured to the leg with three or four removable Velcro straps for 4 weeks. The patients are encouraged to continue to bear weight on the operated limb and to progress gradually to full weight bearing, if they are not doing so already. A trained physiotherapist supervises gentle mobilization exercises of the ankle, isometric contraction of the gastrosoleus complex, and gentle concentric contraction of the calf muscles. Patients are encouraged to perform mobilization of the involved ankle several times per day after unstrapping of the relevant Velcro straps. Patients are reviewed 6 weeks from the operation, when the anterior slab is removed. Stationary cycling and swimming is recommended from the second week after removal of the cast. We allow return to gentle training 6 weeks after removal of the cast. Gradual progression to full sports activity at 20 to 24 weeks from the operation is planned, according to the patient's progress. Resumption of competition is dependent on the patient's plans, but is not recommended before 6 months after surgery. Patients are reviewed at 3, 6, and 9 months from the operation, and every 6 months thereafter. Patients are advised to contact the operating surgeon should any problems ensue. Further physiotherapy, along the lines as described above, is prescribed if symptoms are still present; the patients are followed until they improve, and therefore, are discharged; need further surgery; or default.

Discussion

There has been significant progress in our understanding of Achilles insertional tendinopathy since Clain and Baxter [1] divided Achilles tendon disorders into noninsertional and insertional tendinopathy in 1992. Achilles insertional tendinopathy is a degenerative, rather than an inflammatory, lesion, although the accompanying bursitis may paint a picture of an inflammatory lesion.

The true incidence of Achilles insertional tendinopathy is not clear. Incidence varies from 5% to the most common presentation in athletes. Achilles insertional tendinopathy is recognized as being distinct from retrocalcaneal bursitis and Haglund's deformity, although they often can coexist. Further epidemiologic studies are needed, with a clear terminology, to identify the true incidence of this problem.

The in vitro biomechanical studies on the distal Achilles tendon have given us new insight into possible etiologies. Eccentric calf muscle training was not beneficial in Achilles insertional tendinopathy [16]. This reiterates the fact that the treatment strategies should be different in insertional and noninsertional tendinopathy of the Achilles tendon, because their etiologies are likely to be different. The in vitro strain studies on the distal Achilles tendon identified that the anterior portion of the Achilles insertion is stress-shielded or is underused. This stress-shielded area could be a site for primary degenerative lesion, or could be predisposed to injury because of pre-existing weakness. This can explain the occurrence of this lesion in older, less athletic, overweight individuals, and persons with poor warm-up and stretching habits, and a recent increase in training.

The diagnosis mainly is clinical and radiographs help to confirm the diagnosis as do ultrasound scan or MRI scan. Newer management measures will be introduced as the etiology of Achilles insertional tendinopathy becomes clearer. Various surgical techniques are aimed at debriding the degenerate area of the Achilles tendon; this is accompanied by excision of the retrocalcaneal bursa and resection of the superior prominence. We prefer to reattach the Achilles tendon using bone anchors if one third or more of the Achilles tendon insertion is disinserted.

References

[1] Clain MR, Baxter DE. Achilles tendinitis. Foot Ankle 1992;13(8):482–7.
[2] Astrom M, Rausing A. Chronic Achilles tendinopathy. A survey of surgical and histopathologic findings. Clin Orthop 1995;316:151–64.
[3] Paavola M, Orava S, Leppilahti J, et al. Chronic Achilles tendon overuse injury: complications after surgical treatment. An analysis of 432 consecutive patients. Am J Sports Med 2000;28(1): 77–82.
[4] Benazzo F, Todesca A, Ceciliani L. Achilles tendon tendonitis and heel pain. Oper Tech Sports Med 1997;4(3):179–88.
[5] Kvist M. Achilles tendon injuries in athletes. Sports Med 1994;18(3):173–201.
[6] Myerson MS, McGarvey W. Disorders of the Achilles tendon insertion and Achilles tendinitis. Instr Course Lect 1999;48:211–8.
[7] Schepsis AA, Jones H, Haas AL. Achilles tendon disorders in athletes. Am J Sports Med 2002;30(2):287–305.
[8] Maffulli N, Khan KM, Puddu G. Overuse tendon conditions: time to change a confusing terminology. Arthroscopy 1998;14(8):840–3.
[9] Maffulli N, Testa V, Capasso G, et al. Calcific insertional Achilles tendinopathy: reattachment with bone anchors. Am J Sports Med 2004;32(1):174–82.
[10] Alexander RM, Bennet-Clark HC. Storage of elastic strain energy in muscle and other tissues. Nature 1977;265:114–7.
[11] Fowler A, Philip JF. Abnormality of the calcaneus as a cause of painful heel. Its diagnosis and operative treatment. Br J Surg 1945;32:494–8.
[12] Milz S, Rufai A, Buettner A, et al. Three-dimensional reconstructions of the Achilles tendon insertion in man. J Anat 2002;200(2):145–52.
[13] Merkel KHH, Hess H, Kunz M. Insertion tendinopathy in athletes. A light microscopic, histochemical and electron microscopic examination. Path Res Pract 1982;173:303–9.

[14] Benjamin M, Rufai A, Ralphs JR. The mechanism of formation of bony spurs (enthesophytes) in the Achilles tendon. Arthritis Rheum 2000;43(3):576–83.

[15] Lyman J, Weinhold PS, Almekinders LC. Strain behavior of the distal Achilles tendon: implications for insertional Achilles tendinopathy. Am J Sports Med 2004;32(2):457–61.

[16] Rufai A, Ralphs JR, Benjamin M. Structure and histopathology of the insertional region of the human Achilles tendon. J Orthop Res 1995;13(4):585–93.

[17] Benjamin M, Evans EJ, Copp L. The histology of tendon attachments to bone in man. J Anat 1986;149:89–100.

[18] Wilson AM, Goodship AE. Exercise-induced hyperthermia as a possible mechanism for tendon degeneration. J Biomech 1994;27(7):899–905.

[19] Morris KL, Giacopelli JA, Granoff D. Classification of radiopaque lesions of tendo Achillis. J Foot Surg 1990;29(6):533–42.

[20] Paavola M, Kannus P, Paakkala T, et al. Long-term prognosis of patients with achilles tendinopathy. An observational 8-year follow-up study. Am J Sports Med 2000;28(5):634–42.

[21] Clement DB, Taunton JE, Smart GW. Achilles tendinitis and peritendinitis: etiology and treatment. Am J Sports Med 1984;12(3):179–84.

[22] Almekinders LC. Breaking with tradition. Rehab Manag 2002;15(6):40–2, 45.

[23] Astrom M, Westlin N. No effect of piroxicam on Achilles tendinopathy. A randomized study of 70 patients. Acta Orthop Scand 1992;63(6):631–4.

[24] Marsolais D, Cote CH, Frenette J. Nonsteroidal anti-inflammatory drug reduces neutrophil and macrophage accumulation but does not improve tendon regeneration. Lab Invest 2003;83(7): 991–9.

[25] Fahlstrom M, Jonsson P, Lorentzon R, et al. Chronic Achilles tendon pain treated with eccentric calf-muscle training. Knee Surg Sports Traumatol Arthrosc 2003;11(5):327–33.

[26] Gerken P, McGarvey WC, Baxter DE. Insertional Achilles tendinitis. Foot Ankle Clin N Am 1996;1(112):237–48.

[27] Ohberg L, Alfredson H. Sclerosing therapy in chronic Achilles tendon insertional pain-results of a pilot study. Knee Surg Sports Traumatol Arthrosc 2003;11(5):339–43.

[28] Anderson DL, Taunton JE, Davidson RG. Surgical management of chronic Achilles tendonitis. Clin J Sport Med 1992;2(1):39–42.

[29] Calder JD, Saxby TS. Surgical treatment of insertional Achilles tendinosis. Foot Ankle Int 2003;24(2):119–21.

[30] Kolodziej P, Glisson RR, Nunley JA. Risk of avulsion of the Achilles tendon after partial excision for treatment of insertional tendonitis and Haglund's deformity: a biomechanical study. Foot Ankle Int 1999;20(7):433–7.

[31] McGarvey WC, Palumbo RC, Baxter DE, et al. Insertional Achilles tendinosis: surgical treatment through a central tendon splitting approach. Foot Ankle Int 2002;23(1):19–25.

[32] Watson AD, Anderson RB, Davis WH. Comparison of results of retrocalcaneal decompression for retrocalcaneal bursitis and insertional Achilles tendinosis with calcific spur. Foot Ankle Int 2000;21(8):638–42.

[33] Den Hartog BD. Flexor hallucis longus transfer for chronic Achilles tendonosis. Foot Ankle Int 2003;24(3):233–7.

[34] Leitze Z, Sella EJ, Aversa JM. Endoscopic decompression of the retrocalcaneal space. J Bone Joint Surg Am 2003;85-A(8):1488–96.

[35] Testa V, Maffulli N, Capasso G, et al. Percutaneous longitudinal tenotomy in chronic Achilles tendonitis. Bull Hosp Jt Dis 1996;54:241–4.

ELSEVIER
SAUNDERS

Foot Ankle Clin N Am
10 (2005) 321–329

FOOT AND
ANKLE CLINICS

Conservative Management of Achilles Tendinopathy: New Ideas

Håkan Alfredson, MD, PhD

*Sports Medicine Unit, Department of Surgical and Perioperative Science, Umeå University,
901 87 Umeå, Sweden*

Chronic painful conditions in the Achilles tendon are common, especially among middle-aged recreational athletes [1]. The etiology and pathogenesis are unknown. An association with overuse from repetitive loading is most often considered the main etiologic factor [2–4]; however, these conditions also are seen in nonathletic individuals [5,6]. In 342 patients who had chronic Achilles tendinopathy, physical activity was not correlated to the histopathology; this suggested that physical activity could be more important in provoking the symptoms than being the cause of the actual lesion [7]. Other suggested etiologic factors are ageing with a decreased blood supply and decreased tensile strength, muscle weakness and imbalance, and insufficient flexibility [8–12]. There is a wide range of suggested etiologic factors; the scientific background of most of these suggestions is lacking and they should be characterized as nonproven theories.

A correct clinical diagnosis can be established by clinical examination, combined with ultrasonography [13–15], MRI [13–15], or biopsy [16]. Patients who have Achilles tendinopathy commonly present with morning stiffness in the tendon, and a gradual onset of pain during tendon-loading activity [6,17,18]. Most often, clinical examination reveals tenderness, and often, but not always, a localized swelling in the tendon. It is important to exclude other conditions, such as os trigonum syndrome, tenosynovitis or dislocation of the peroneal tendons, tenosynovitis of the plantar flexors, an accessory soleus muscle, tumors of the Achilles tendon (xanthomas), and neuroma of the suralis nerve. Hypoechoic areas on ultrasound and areas with increased signal intensity on MRI correspond to areas of altered collagen fiber structure and increased interfibrillar ground substance (hydrophilic glycosamino-glycans) [5]. The combination of chronic

E-mail address: hakan.alfredson@idrott.umu.se

pain symptoms from a tender area in the midportion of the Achilles tendon, and corresponding changes in the tendon at imaging, gives rise to the clinical syndrome of chronic Achilles tendinopathy [5,18]. This article gives an update on recently developed conservative treatment methods for the management of chronic Achilles tendinopathy.

Conservative treatment methods

Background

There are few scientific prospective studies, and few studies that compared different types of conservative management regimens for the chronic painful Achilles tendon in a randomized manner. Conservative management is recommended as the initial strategy [1,2,4,6,8–10,18–20], with identification and correction of possible etiologic factors, at times using a symptom-related approach.

Training errors, [8,11,21,22], muscle weakness [2,4,23–25], decreased flexibility [2,4,8,9,26–28], biomechanical "abnormalities" [8,9,11], and poor equipment [19,21,29] have been suggested as important etiologic factors. Again, these suggestions are based on poor scientific grounds and are to be considered unsubstantiated hypotheses.

Despite the absence of scientific evidence for an ongoing chemical inflammation inside the tendon [6,18,24], nonsteroidal anti-inflammatory drugs (NSAIDs) are used often as one part of the initial management [8,9,11,26,30–33]. Consequently, the use of NSAIDs with the purpose to diminish chemical inflammation in the chronic painful Achilles tendon can be questioned. In a randomized, double-blind, placebo-controlled study of 70 patients who had chronic painful Achilles tendinopathy, oral piroxicam gave similar results as placebo [34].

Management with corticosteroid injections is being debated [4,35,36]. Most investigators suggest that corticosteroid injections should be placed outside the tendon to avoid damage to the tendon tissue, but there are groups that suggest intratendinous injections [37,38]. Partial ruptures are found after steroid injections [7,12,39,40] and management with steroid injections were shown to predict a partial rupture in patients who had chronic Achilles tendinopathy [7]. Also, a large number of patients who are operated on for chronic Achilles tendinopathy had received corticosteroid injections; this indicates a poor effect of corticosteroids.

Modalities, such cold therapy [9], heat [41], massage [42], ultrasound [43], electrical stimulation [44], and laser therapy [45] sometimes are included in the management regimen. These modalities are reported to be effective, but, to the best of the author's knowledge, no well-planned scientific clinical study has confirmed their effects.

The initial management most commonly consists of a multi-oriented approach, with combined rehabilitation models. There are many different designs, most often including a combination of rest (complete or modified), medication

(NSAIDs, corticosteroids), orthotics (heel lift, change of shoes, corrections of malalignments), stretching and massage, and strength training [2,4,8,9,11,12,20].

Recently developed management models

The importance of eccentric training as a part of the rehabilitation of tendon injuries was stressed in the early 1980s by Curvin and Stanish [2]. Using their approach, we designed an eccentric calf muscle training regimen to be used on a well-defined diagnosis. We decided to try this model on patients who had chronic painful midportion Achilles tendinopathy, because the midportion of the Achilles tendon is an area that can be examined easily clinically and by ultrasound or MRI. First, in a prospective pilot study on recreational athletes, we reported good clinical short-term results with painful eccentric calf-muscle training [19]. All 15 patients in that study had localized changes at 2 cm to 6 cm from the insertion of the tendon into the calcaneus; this corresponded to the painful area that was verified with ultrasonography. In all patients, conventional management (rest, NSAIDs, change of shoes, orthoses, pain-free muscular training) had been tried without effects, and all patients were on the waiting list

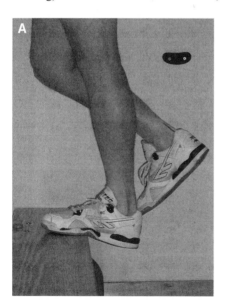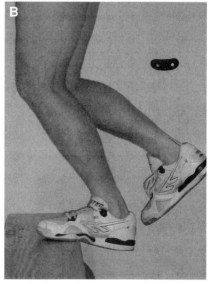

Fig. 1. From an upright body position and standing with all body weight on the ventral half of the foot, with the ankle joint in plantarflexion and lifted by the noninjured leg, the calf muscle is loaded eccentrically by having the patient lower the heel beneath the lever. Eccentric calf muscle loading with the knee straight (*A*), and to maximize the activation of the soleus muscle, eccentric calf muscle loading with the knee bent (*B*). When the exercises can be done without experiencing pain in the tendon, the load should be increased to reach a new level of "painful training" by using a backpack that is filled gradually with weights, or by using a weight machine (*C*). (*From* Alfredson H. Chronic midportion Achilles tendinopathy: an update on research and treatment. Clin Sports Med 2003;22(4):736.)

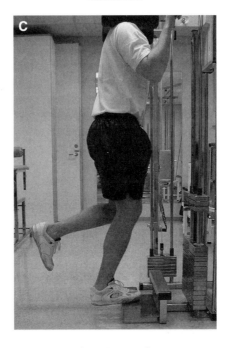

Fig. 1 (*continued*).

for surgery. The patients performed three sets of 15 eccentric heel drops (Fig. 1) twice a day, 7 days a week, for 12 weeks. This type of eccentric tendon loading is painful, and the patients were told to continue their exercises despite experiencing pain or discomfort at or around the tendon. The exercises were supposed to be painful; if there was no tendon pain during the exercise, the load was increased gradually to reach "a new level of painful training." After 12 weeks, all 15 patients were satisfied and were back to their preinjury activity levels. No patient underwent surgery. The pain score (visual analog scale) during activity (running) decreased from an average of 81.2 before the eccentric training regimen to 4.8 after training. Follow-ups showed that only one patient needed surgical management as a result of the recurrence of Achilles tendon pain. The other 14 patients remain satisfied with the result of management. At our institution, we routinely manage patients who have a diagnosis of chronic Achilles tendinopathy of the main body of the tendon with this type of painful training; follow-up showed satisfactory results in 90 of 101 tendons [46]. From that study, patients who had chronic insertional Achilles tendon pain showed a satisfactory result after painful eccentric training in only 10 of 31 tendons. Consequently, eccentric training has a poor potential for management of chronic pain in the Achilles tendon insertion.

Secondly, to find out whether painful concentric calf muscle training also could give a good clinical result, we performed a randomized, prospective, multi-center study; patients who had painful chronic tendinopathy of the main body of the Achilles tendon were randomized to concentric or eccentric training [47]. The eccentric training program was the same as previously described [19], whereas the concentric training program was designed to include exercises that contained mainly concentric calf muscle action. For both programs, training was encouraged, despite experiencing pain or discomfort in the tendon. The eccentric training regimen (81% of patients satisfied and back to previous activity level) produced significantly better clinical results than the concentric training regimen (38% satisfied patients) [47].

In a clinical and ultrasonographic (gray-scale ultrasound) follow-up (mean 3.8 years) of patients who underwent eccentric training, most were satisfied and back to previous tendon loading activity level. The Achilles tendon thickness had decreased significantly, and the tendon structure looked more normal ultrasonographically in the successfully treated cases [48].

We cannot explain the background to the good clinical results that were achieved with painful eccentric calf muscle training. Relief of pain may result from the increased tensile strength in the tendon, or, possibly, from stretching with "lengthening" of the muscle–tendon unit, and consequently, less strain during ankle joint motion. Also, the eccentric training regimen is painful to perform; this type of painful loading may be associated with some kind of alteration of the pain perception from the tendon. The findings using grey-scale ultrasonography together with color Doppler have added important information that may explain how and why the eccentric training regimen works. In a study that used ultrasonography and color Doppler, we recently showed that in Achilles tendons with chronic painful tendinopathy—but not in normal pain-free tendons—there is neovascularization outside and inside the ventral part of the tendinopathic area [49]. Using ultrasonography and color Doppler during eccentric calf muscle contraction, the flow in the neovessels disappeared when the ankle was dorsiflexed. These observations raised the question if the good clinical effects that are demonstrated with eccentric training could be due to action on the neovessels, and whether the neovessels and accompanying nerves were the main source of pain. In a recent study, ultrasound and color Doppler follow-up showed that most patients with good clinical results had no residual neovessels. Patients with a poor result showed residual neovascularization [50]. These findings indicate that the area with neovessels may be important for the pain that is suffered during Achilles tendon loading activity.

In a further study, we injected a local anesthetic in the area with neovessels outside the tendon [51]. This resulted in a pain-free tendon; patients could load their Achilles tendon without experiencing any pain from the tendon. From these findings, we hypothesized that the neovessels and accompanying nerves were responsible for the pain in the tendinopathy area. To test this hypothesis, in a noncontrolled pilot study, we injected a sclerosing agent (Polidocanol) in the area with neovessels on the ventral side of the tendon (Fig. 2). The short-term (6 months) results were promising; 8 of 10 patients were pain-free and satisfied with the management after a mean of two injections [52]. At 6 months, the successfully treated patients showed no neovessels outside or inside the tendon.

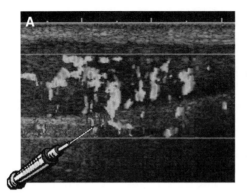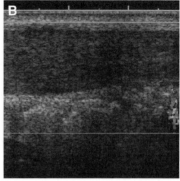

Fig. 2. Grey-scale ultrasonography and color Doppler examination (longitudinal view) of tendinopathy of the main body of the Achilles tendon. The affected area is thick, irregular, and echo poor. There is a neovascularization outside and inside the ventral part of the area with tendon changes. (*A*) Before injection of the sclerosing substance. Note the position of the needle close to the neovessels outside the anterior part of the tendon. (*B*) After injection. Note that there are no residual neovessels.

In the 2 patients who did not have a successful outcome, residual neovessels were still present. At 2 years (unpublished data), the same 8 patients were satisfied and pain-free, and there were no residual neovessels in the tendon. Also, the tendon thickness had decreased, and ultrasonographically the tendon structure looked more normal. The results of this new intervention are promising, but longer follow-ups of clinical status and sonographic findings are needed for further evaluation. The results of a randomized controlled study that compared the effects of injections of a sclerosing and a nonsclerosing substance are under evaluation.

We used ultrasonography combined with color Doppler to investigate the chronic painful Achilles tendon insertion. In the area of the tendon insertion, the tendon, bursae, and bone, alone or together, may be responsible for the pain. This condition also shows localized neovascularization, with vessels coming anteriorly, sometimes in close relation to the walls of the retrocalcaneal bursa, and cruising into the distal tendon. In a pilot study, we tried sclerosing injections on this condition [53]. The results showed that 8 of 11 patients were satisfied with the intervention and were back to previous tendon-loading activity level. Seven of the 8 satisfied patients showed no residual neovascularization. Two of the three patients with a poor result had bony spurs. Again, the results are promising, but more patients with different activity levels and different sonographic findings need to be studied before more definitive conclusions can be drawn. It is likely that patients who also have severe bone pathology, and thereby mechanical problems, are less suitable for this type of intervention.

Rehabilitation after sclerosing injections includes a short period of rest (1–3 days), then gradually increased tendon-loading activities, but no maximum loading (jumping, fast runs, heavy strength training) for the first 2 weeks. After 2 weeks, maximum tendon loading is allowed. After treating 150 patients who had Achilles tendinopathy with sclerosing injections, we had two complications that may be related to this regimen. One patient who had insertion Achilles tendinopathy sustained a total rupture in the proximal part of the tendon at the end of an 800-m running race, and one patient sustained a partial rupture in a midportion of the tendon where he previously had received four intratendinous corticosteroid injections.

Summary

Chronic Achilles tendinopathy is difficult to treat, and results, even after surgical management, are variable. The few studies that reported long-term results indicated a poor outcome. Also, surgery requires prolonged rehabilitation, and, depending on the patient's occupation, a varying period of sick leave from work. For tendinopathy of the main body of the Achilles tendon, painful eccentric calf muscle training gave good short- to mid-term results, and does not require taking sick leave from work. Sclerosing injections that target the area with neovessels and nerves outside the tendon gives promising results in the midportion and in the Achilles tendon insertion, but needs further scientific evaluation before its general use can be recommended.

References

[1] Kvist M. Achilles tendon injuries in athletes. Sports Med 1994;18(3):173–201.

[2] Curvin S, Stanish WD. Tendinitis: its etiology and treatment. Lexington (KY): Collamore Press, DC Heath & Co.; 1984.

[3] Archambault JM, Wiley P, Bray RC. Exercise loading of tendons and the development of overuse injuries. A review. Sports Med 1995;20(2):77–89.

[4] Józsa LG, Kannus P. Human tendons. Anatomy, physiology, and pathology. Champaign, IL: Human Kinetics Publishers; 1997. p. 1–573.

[5] Movin T. Aspects of aetiology, pathoanatomy and diagnostic methods in chronic mid-portion Achillodynia [doctoral dissertation]. Stockholm (Sweden): Karolinska Institute Stockholm; 1998.

[6] Alfredson H, Lorentzon R. Chronic Achilles tendinosis. Recommendations for treatment and prevention. Sports Med 2000;29(2):135–46.

[7] Åström M. Partial rupture in chronic Achilles tendinopathy. A retrospective analysis of 342 cases. Acta Orthop Scand 1998;69(4):404–7.

[8] Welsh RP, Clodman J. Clinical survey of Achilles tendinitis in athletes. Can Med Assoc J 1980;122:193–5.

[9] Clement DB, Taunton JE, Smart GW. Achilles tendinitis and peritendinitis: etiology and treatment. Am J Sports Med 1984;12:179–84.

[10] Nichols AW. Achilles tendinitis in running athletes. J Am Board Fam Pract 1989;2:196–203.

[11] James SL, Bates BT, Osternig LR. Injuries to runners. Am J Sports Med 1978;6(2):40–50.

[12] Galloway MT, Jokl P, Dayton OW. Achilles tendon overuse injuries. Clin Sports Med 1992; 11(4):771–82.

[13] Åström M, Gentz CF, Nilsson P, et al. Imaging in chronic Achilles tendinopathy: a comparison of ultrasonography, magnetic resonance imaging and surgical findings in 27 histologically verified cases. Skeletal Radiol 1996;25:615–20.

[14] Paavola M, Paakkala T, Kannus P, et al. Ultrasonography in the differential diagnosis of Achilles tendon injuries and related disorders. Acta Radiol 1998;39:612–9.

[15] Neuhold A, Stiskal M, Kainberger F, et al. Degenerative Achilles tendon disease: assessment by magnetic resonance and ultrasonography. Eur J Radiol 1992;14:213–20.

[16] Movin T, Gad A, Reinholt FP. Tendon pathology in long-standing Achillodynia. Biopsy findings in 40 patients. Acta Orthop Scand 1997;68(2):170–5.

[17] Åström M. On the nature and etiology of chronic Achilles tendinopathy [doctoral dissertation]. Lund (Sweden): University of Lund; 1997.

[18] Khan KM, Cook JL, Bonar F, et al. Histopathology of common tendinopathies. Update and implications for clinical management. Sports Med 1999;27(6):393–408.

[19] Alfredson H, Pietilä T, Jonsson P, et al. Heavy-load eccentric calf muscle training for the treatment of chronic Achilles tendinosis. Am J Sports Med 1998;26(3):360–6.

[20] Sandmeier R, Renström PAFH. Diagnosis and treatment of chronic tendon disorders in sports. Scand J Med Sci Sports 1997;7:96–106.

[21] Brody DM. Running injuries. Prevention and management. Clin Symp 1987;39:1–36.

[22] Clancy Jr WG. Tendinitis and plantar fascitis in runners. In: D'Ambrosia R, Drez Jr D, editors. Prevention and treatment of running injuries. Thorofare, NJ: Charles B Slack, Inc.; 1982.

[23] Appel H-J. Skeletal muscle atrophy during immobilization. Int J Sports Med 1986;7:1–5.

[24] Renström PAFH. Diagnosis and management of overuse injuries. In: Dirix A, Knuttgen HG, Tiitel K, editors. The Olympic book of sports medicine, vol 1. Oxford (UK): Blackwell Scientific Publications; 1988. p. 446–68.

[25] Nicol C, Komi PV, Marconnet F. Fatigue effects of marathon running on neuromuscular performance. II: changes in force, integrated electromyographic activity and endurance capacity. Scand J Med Sci Sports 1991;1:10–7.

[26] Kvist M. Achilles tendon injuries in athletes. Ann Chir Gynaecol 1991;80:188–201.

[27] Leach RE, Dilorio E, Harney RA. Pathologic hindfoot conditions in the athlete. Clin Orthop 1983;177:116–21.

[28] Wallin D, Ekblom B, Grahn R, et al. Improvement of muscle flexibility. A comparison between two techniques. Am J Sports Med 1985;13:263–8.

[29] Jörgensen U, Ekstrand J. Significance of heel pad confinement for the shock absorption at heel strike. Int J Sports Med 1988;9:468–73.

[30] Leppilahti J, Orava S, Karpakka J, et al. Overuse injuries of the Achilles tendon. Ann Chir Gynaecol 1991;80:202–7.

[31] Teitz CC, Garrett Jr WE, Miniaci A, et al. Tendon problems in athletic individuals. J Bone Joint Surg Am 1997;79:138–52.

[32] Weiler JM. Medical modifiers of sports injury. The use of nonsteroidal anti-inflammatory drugs (NSAIDs) in sports soft-tissue injury. Clin Sports Med 1992;11:625–44.

[33] Saltzman CL, Tearse DS. Achilles tendon injuries. J Am Acad Orthop Surg 1998;6:316–25.

[34] Åström M, Westlin N. No effect of piroxicam on Achilles tendinopathy. A randomized study of 70 patients. Acta Orthop Scand 1992;63:631–4.

[35] Leadbetter WB. Anti-inflammatory therapy and sports injury: The role of non-steroidal drugs and corticosteroid injection. Clin Sports Med 1995;14:353–410.

[36] Schrier I, Matheson GO, Kohl III HW. Achilles tendonitis: are corticosteroid injections useful or harmful? Clin J Sport Med 1996;6(4):245–50.

[37] Koenig MJ, Torp-Pedersen S, Qvistgaard E, et al. Preliminary results of colour Doppler-guided intratendinous glucocorticoid injection for Achilles tendonitis in five patients. Scand J Med Sci Sports 2004;14(2):100–6.

[38] Fredberg U, Bolvig L, Pfeiffer-Jensen M, et al. Ultrasonography as a tool for diagnosis, guidance of local steroid injection and, together with pressure algometry, monitoring of the treatment of athletes with chronic jumper's knee and Achilles tendinitis: a randomized, double blind, placebo-controlled study. Scand J Rheumatol 2004;33(2):94–101.

[39] Williams JGP. Achilles tendon lesions in sport. Sports Med 1986;3:114–35.

[40] Ljungqvist R. Subcutaneous partial rupture of the Achilles tendon. Acta Orthop Scand 1968; (Suppl 113):1–86.

[41] Houglum PA. Soft tissue healing and its impact on rehabilitation. J Sport Rehabil 1992;1: 19–39.

[42] Rogoff JB, editor. Manipulation, traction, and massage. 2nd edition. Baltimore (MD): Williams & Williams; 1989.

[43] Prentice WE, Malone TR. Thermotherapy. In: Leadbetter WB, Buchwalther JA, Gordon SL, editors. Sports-induced inflammation. Park Ridge: AAOS; 1990. p. 455–61.

[44] Rivenburgh DW. Physical modalities in the treatment of tendon injuries. Clin Sports Med 1992;11:645–59.

[45] Siebert W, Seichert N, Sieben B, et al. What is the efficacy of 'soft' and 'mid' lasers in therapy of tendinopathies? A double-blind study. Arch Orthop Trauma Surg 1987;106:358–63.

[46] Fahlström M, Jonsson P, Lorentzon R, et al. Chronic Achilles tendon pain treated with eccentric calf-muscle training. Knee Surg Sports Traumatol Arthrosc 2003;11:327–33.

[47] Mafi N, Lorentzon R, Alfredson H. Superior results with eccentric calf-muscle training compared to concentric training in a randomized prospective multi-center study on patients with chronic Achilles tendinosis. Knee Surg Sports Traumatol Arthrosc 2001;9:42–7.

[48] Öhberg L, Lorentzon R, Alfredson H. Eccentric training in patients with chronic Achilles tendinosis: normalised tendon structure and decreased thickness at follow up. Br J Sports Med 2004;38:8–11.

[49] Öhberg L, Lorentzon R, Alfredson H. Neovascularisation in Achilles tendons with painful tendinosis but not in normal tendons: an ultrasonographic investigation. Knee Surg Sports Traumatol Arthrosc 2001;9:233–8.

[50] Öhberg L, Alfredson H. Effects on neovascularisation behind the good results with eccentric training in chronic mid-portion Achilles tendinosis? Knee Surg Sports Traumatol Arthrosc 2004;12:465–70.

[51] Alfredson H, Öhberg L, Forsgren S. Is vasculo-neural ingrowth the cause of pain in chronic Achilles tendinosis? An investigation using ultrasonography and colour Doppler, immunohistochemistry, and diagnostic injections. Knee Surg Sports Traumatol Arthrosc 2003;11:334–8.

[52] Öhberg L, Alfredson H. Ultrasound guided sclerosing of neovessels in painful chronic Achilles tendinosis: pilot study of a new treatment. Br J Sports Med 2002;36:173–7.

[53] Öhberg L, Alfredson H. Sclerosing therapy in chronic Achilles tendon insertional pain-results of a pilot study. Knee Surg Sports Traumatol Arthrosc 2003;11:339–43.

ELSEVIER
SAUNDERS

Foot Ankle Clin N Am
10 (2005) 331–356

FOOT AND
ANKLE CLINICS

Acute Rupture of the Achilles Tendon

Tomas Movin, MD, PhD[a], Åsa Ryberg, MD[a],
Donald J. McBride, FRCS(Orth)[b],
Nicola Maffulli, MD, MS, PhD, FRCS(Orth)[b],*

[a]*Department of Orthopaedics, Huddinge Hospital, Karolinska Institute, S-14186, Stockholm, Sweden*
[b]*Department of Trauma and Orthopaedics, Keele University School of Medicine, Thornburrow Drive,
Hartshill, Stoke-on-Trent ST4 7QB, UK*

Acute subcutaneous Achilles tendon ruptures are increasingly frequent, mainly because of the greater participation in recreational sports by the general population that alternates exercise with inactivity [1]. Its etiology is multifactorial, and its true nature remains unclear. The diagnosis of an acute Achilles tendon rupture can be made on history and physical examination, without the adjunct of imaging [2].

The best management method of the acute Achilles tendon rupture is controversial and debated (Table 1) [3]. Treatment can be classified broadly into surgical (open repair or percutaneous repair) and nonsurgical (cast immobilization or functional bracing) types. Postoperative splintage can be with a rigid cast (above or below the knee) or a functional brace. Open surgical repair of an acute Achilles tendon rupture significantly reduces the risk of rerupture compared with nonsurgical treatment, but has a significantly greater risk of other complications, including wound infection. The risk of wound infection can be reduced by performing surgery percutaneously. Postoperative splintage in a functional brace seems to reduce time off from work and sports, and may decrease the overall complication rate. The management of uncomplicated acute Achilles tendon ruptures should be individualized according to the concerns, occupation, sports participation, and health of the patient [3].

---

* Corresponding author.
E-mail address: n.maffulli@keele.ac.uk (N. Maffulli).

1083-7515/05/$ – see front matter © 2005 Elsevier Inc. All rights reserved.
doi:10.1016/j.fcl.2005.01.003

Table 1
Review articles that compared surgical and nonsurgical treatment of Achilles tendon rupture

Author and year of publication	Number of articles included (number of Achilles tendon ruptures)	Nonsurgical complication rate	Nonsurgical rerupture rate	Surgical complication rate	Surgical rerupture rate
Wills et al, 1986 [4]	20 (1003)	2/20 (10%)	40/226 (17.7%)	155/777 (19.9%)	12/777 (1.5%)
Cetti et al, 1993 [5]	66 (4597)	24/514 (4.7%)	69/514 (13.4%)	425/4083 (10.4%)	58/4083 (1.4%)
Lo et al, 1997 [6]	19 (990)	10/248 (4%)	29/248 (11.7%)	196/742 (26.4%)	21/742 (2.8%)
Popovic & Lemaire, 1999 [7]	16 (5046)	27/569 (4.7%)	76/569 (13.3%)	492/4477 (11.0%)	69/4477 (1.5%)
Wong et al, 2002 [3]	125 (5056)	62/645 (9.6%)	63/645 (9.8%)	976/4411 (22.1%)	103/4411 (2.3%)
Bhandari et al, 2002 [8]	6 (448)	0/210 (0%)[a]	29/233 (12.4%)	10/211 (4.7%)	7/225 (3.1%)
Kocher et al, 2002 [9]	32 (1893)	12/365 (3.3%)	29/347 (8.4%)	306/1487 (20.6%)	32/1437 (2.2%)
Khan et al, 2004 [10]	4 (356)	5/183 (2.7%)	23/183 (12.6%)	59/173 (34.1%)	6/173 (3.5%)

[a] Limited to infection.

Basic anatomy and biomechanics

The Achilles tendon transmits the tension that is generated by the gastrocnemius and soleus muscles to the os calcis. The former muscle arises with two muscle bellies from the posterior aspect of the femoral condyles, whereas the latter arises from the upper end of the tibial and fibular posterior surfaces. The tendon aponeurosis from the three muscles bellies join to form the common tendon. The gastrocnemius component of the Achilles tendon is 11 cm to 26 cm long; the soleus component is 3 cm to 11 cm long [11]. During its course to its insertion on the calcaneal tuberosity, the fibers rotate 90° so that those that are located medially proximally become posterior distally [11,12]. At the calcaneal tuberosity, the tendon fibers diverge to insert over the dorsal aspect of the calcaneus. The insertion part is composed of the attachment of the tendon, a layer of hyaline cartilage, and an area of bone that is not covered by periosteum [13].

The tendon is able to transmit forces from the contracting muscles to the bone and can deform and recover its original length if the strain does not exceed approximately 4% [14]. Thereby, the tendon is shock absorbent and protects the muscles from damage; however, if the strains are between 4% and 8%, the tendon fibers are damaged and the collagen fibers start to slide past one another as the intermolecular cross-links fail. At a strain level of approximately 8%, the Achilles tendon ultimately ruptures. Eccentric muscle actions put the tendon under highest stress [15]. Typically, heavy loading, high-speed eccentric muscle actions that involve the calf muscles and the Achilles tendon are the transition to fast push-off during running or sudden dorsiflexion at the ankle joint. Further, the Achilles tendon can be subjected to nonuniform stresses through modifications of individual muscle contributions. An injury, therefore, can be produced by a discrepancy in individual muscle forces that are caused, for example, by asynchronous contraction of the various components of the triceps surae or by uncoordinated agonist–antagonist muscle contraction that is due to impaired transmission of peripheral sensory stimuli [16].

The age of the individual and the size of the tendon are important factors for the biomechanical properties of the Achilles tendon and its capability to cope with the high stress levels. Younger individuals have significantly higher tensile rupture stress and lower stiffness [17]; increased age, body height, cross-sectional calf muscle size, and foot size correlate significantly with thicker Achilles tendons [18]. The Achilles tendon's cross-sectional area is larger in runners than in nonrunners [19], and in elderly athletes than in elderly sedentary men [20]. This suggests that chronic exposure of the Achilles tendon to loading results in tendon adaptation in man that is on par with exercise-induced tendon hypertrophy in animal models [21–24].

Strength training of the calf muscles produces a 12% to 17% increase in the volume of the Achilles tendon within 30 minutes [25]. This increase may be explained by a higher water content or hyperemia in the Achilles tendon. This immediate response and adaptation to exercise may affect Achilles tendon stiffness and modulus. Theoretically, an increase in tendon volume would yield greater stiffness for a given deformation, with changes in the intratendinous biomechanical properties.

The Achilles tendon receives its blood supply from three regions—the musculotendinous junction, along its length, and in the region of insertion [26–28]. Anteriorly, vessels can enter the tendon through a mesotenon [27]. In the tendon itself, vessels in the endotenon run longitudinally between the collagen bundles. The density of vessels was reported to be lowest in the midportion of the tendon as assessed by angiographic injection techniques [28,29] and vessel density measurements on histologic material [30,31]. Conversely, the blood flow that was assessed by laser Doppler flowmetry in vivo in healthy volunteers was significantly less at the calcaneal insertion, but was distributed evenly in the midportion and the musculotendinous junction. The blood flow in the tendon depends on age, with a greater blood flow in younger individuals [32] and under loading conditions [33,34].

Epidemiology

Achilles tendon rupture usually occurs in middle-aged men who work in a white-collar profession during sports activities [35]. Its incidence has increased during the last decades, at least in northern Europe and Scotland [1,36–42]. Patients who have Achilles tendon rupture can be classified into two subgroups— young or middle-aged athletes and older nonathletes. Epidemiologic data from Malmö, Sweden [36,38] showed an incidence curve with two peaks [38], a larger one in young or middle-aged individuals, and a smaller one in patents in their seventies. Compared with the age-specific incidence in 1950 to 1973, a marked increase in sports and nonathletic injuries was found; patients in the latter group were older than during the earlier period. The increase in the athletic group is explained mostly by increased participation in recreational sports. The cause of the increase in the elderly group is unknown, although 13% of ruptures occur in patients who are older than 65 years [43].

Leppilahti et al [39] found an increased incidence of Achilles tendon ruptures in Oulo, Finland from 2 in 100,000 in 1979 to 1986 to 12 in 100,000 in 1987 to 1994; they also demonstrated a bimodal age distribution. The incidence was greatest in the age group from 30 to 39 years, with a smaller peak incidence between 50 and 59 years. The mean age was significantly less for the sports injuries.

Achilles tendon rupture is predominantly a male disease. The dominance of men is evident in all studies, with a male:female ratio of 2:1 to 12:1; this probably reflects the greater prevalence of men who are involved in sports [1,44–46]. Almost all studies report a dominance of left-sided Achilles tendon ruptures. In a review by Arndt [46], 57% of 1823 Achilles tendon ruptures were left-sided, probably because of the greater prevalence of right-side–dominant individuals who push off with the left lower limb [1,35].

Hungarian and Finnish studies showed a increased prevalence of rupture of the Achilles tendon in patients with blood group O [47,48]. These findings have not been confirmed in another Finnish area and in Scotland [39,49], probably as a result of peculiarities in the distribution of the ABO groups in genetically-segregated populations.

Among U.S. military personnel who underwent repair of Achilles tendon ruptures between 1994 and 1996, blacks were at increased risk for undergoing repair of the Achilles tendon compared with nonblacks [50].

Pathobiomechanics

Achilles tendon ruptures occur commonly in the midsubstance of the tendon, usually 2 cm to 6 cm proximal to the insertion to the calcaneus. Other less common locations are the musculotendinous junction and the insertion into the calcaneus. The injury can be open or closed, and may be caused by a direct blow or an indirect force. Most injuries tend to occur when pushing off with the weight-bearing foot while extending the knee. Some Achilles tendon ruptures occur following sudden ankle dorsiflexion or violent dorsiflexion of a plantar flexed foot [51,52]. Most ruptures occur during sport. The sport that dominates as the cause of Achilles tendon rupture depends on the country in which the study is performed. In the U.S. military, basketball was the most common sport [50]; in Germany; it was soccer [53,54]; and in Scandinavian countries; badminton players present with most of the Achilles tendon ruptures [35,36,38,39,55–58].

Etiology

The exact reason why the Achilles tendon ruptures is not known. Two main theories are advocated: the "degeneration theory" and the "mechanical theory." According to the degeneration theory, chronic degeneration of the tendon leads to a rupture without excessive loads being applied. Degenerative changes can result from several factors, including physiologic alterations in the tendon, chronic overloading with microtrauma, pharmacologic treatment, and in association with other diseases.

Kannus and Jozsa [37] compared the histopathology of 397 Achilles tendon ruptures with 220 control tendons, using conventional and polarized light microscopy and scanning and transmission electron microscopy. A healthy structure was not seen in any spontaneously ruptured tendon; however, two thirds of the control tendons were structurally healthy. There were characteristic histopathologic patterns in the spontaneously ruptured tendons. Most (97%) of the pathologic changes were degenerative, with hypoxic (45%), mucoid (19%), tendolipomatous (6%), and calcifying tendinopathy (3%), alone or in combination. These changes also were found in 31% of the control tendons.

The homeostasis of the extracellular matrix components, such as the fibrillar collagens and the proteoglycans, may be affected and predispose to a rupture. Type I collagen accounts for 95% of collagen in normal tendons. This parallel arrangement imparts high tensile strength to the tendon [59]. Ruptured tendons contain significantly greater proportions of type III collagen and reduced amounts type I collagen, together with significantly higher degrees of degeneration, than nonruptured tendons [59]. Type III collagen is less resistant to tensile forces and may predispose the tendon to spontaneous rupture.

At electron microscopy, ruptured Achilles tendons show a loss of larger collagen fibrils at the rupture site compared with normal tendons [60]. An inverse relationship between the amount of type III collagen and fibril diameter may exist [61]. Versican is the main large proteoglycan that is expressed in the midportion of the Achilles tendon. Corps et al [62] found changes in versican expression relative to that of collagen in ruptured Achilles tendons; further alterations in the balance of versican splice variants may contribute to changes in matrix structure and function.

Decorin, a small proteoglycan that modulates collagen fibrillogenesis, is a vital player in maintaining tendon integrity at the molecular level [63]. The glycosaminoglycans that are bound to decorin act as bridges between contiguous fibrils that connect adjacent fibrils every 64 nm to 68 nm. This architectural arrangement suggests a possible role in providing mechanical integrity of the tendon structure. Laboratory evidence suggests that fluoroquinolone antibiotics decrease decorin transcription [64], which may alter the viscoelastic properties of the tendons and induce increased fragility [65].

Most patients have no symptoms before the rupture. Hence, clinical painful tendinopathy is not a common etiologic factor to complete Achilles tendon ruptures [60]. Nine (5%) of the 176 patients who presented with a rupture of the Achilles tendon in Aberdeen, Scotland between January 1990 and December 1995 had previous symptoms [1]. Nestorson et al [43], however, reported that among 25 patients who had Achilles tendon rupture who were older than 65 years age, 11 (44%) had experienced Achilles tendon symptoms; 7 had received local cortisone injections. Although clinical painful tendinopathy seemingly is a risk factor, patients who had chronic Achilles tendinopathy in reported nonsurgical and surgical series had a long duration of symptoms (several months or years) without sustaining a rupture [66–68]. Conversely, at the time of Achilles tendon rupture, degeneration and necrosis was present in 47 of 50 and 42 of 50 of the contralateral asymptomatic Achilles tendons, respectively. Spontaneous rupture of the Achilles tendon seems to be preceded by widespread, bilateral damage of the tendon [69]. Also, the patients' asymptomatic contralateral Achilles tendons showed a greater prevalence of intratendinous alterations with ultrasonography [70].

Simultaneous bilateral ruptures without preceding factors are rare [71–73], whereas subsequent ruptures on one side after the other has been reported in up to 6% of patients [74].

An Achilles tendon rupture also can result from an adverse drug event. Local and systemic corticosteroids are a risk factor for tendon rupture [75];

fluoroquinolone antibiotics, such as ciprofloxacin, have been implicated in the rupture of the Achilles tendon during the last decade [76,77].

Spontaneous rupture of the Achilles tendon has been associated with a multitude of disorders, such as inflammatory and autoimmune conditions [78], genetically determined collagen abnormalities [79], infectious diseases [51], and hyperlipidemia [80,82].

High serum lipid concentrations have been reported in patients who have complete rupture of the Achilles tendon [80,81]. Although there is uptake and excretion of sterols by the enzyme, sterol 27-hydroxylase (CYP27A1), in the Achilles tendon [82], histopathologic evidence of lipomatosis was found in only 6% of specimens from Achilles tendon ruptures [37]. Further, patients who have familiar hypercholesterolemia and Achilles tendon xanthomata do not seem to be at greater risk of ruptures.

Diagnosis

The history in most cases is typical and does not pose diagnostic problems [2]. The patient suddenly feels a "pop" or "snap" in the calf, and sometimes hears a crack. The patients often believes that had been struck or kicked in the posterior aspect of the distal part of the leg. The immediate pain resolves soon. Persistent weakness, poor balance, and altered gait are common. A direct injury mechanism to the Achilles tendon is rare.

On other occasions, when sports participation is not involved, the injury may be missed or misjudged by the patient or the doctor. Further difficulties in reaching the correct diagnosis may occur in elderly patients or if the patient consults a doctor some days after the injury; Achilles tendon ruptures are missed in up to 25% of patients [83,84]. In elderly patients who have Achilles tendon rupture, 9 (36%) of 25 patients had a delay of more than 1 week to treatment [43].

The diagnosis of Achilles tendon rupture is clinical [2]. Within 2 to 3 days from the injury, a gap can be palpated that is 2 cm to 7 cm proximal to the insertion of the Achilles tendon on the calcaneus. In a surgical series of 303 patients, the average gap was 4.8 cm proximal to the insertion [85]. Later, the gap often is filled with hematoma and fibrous tissue; swelling, edema, and bruising may make palpation more difficult.

Several diagnostic tests have been used. The calf squeeze test and knee flexion test are used without any equipment, and therefore, are recommended highly. If they are positive, the diagnosis is certain [2]. The calf squeeze test, first described by Simmonds in 1957 [86] and 5 years later by Thompson and Doherty [87], is simple and reliable. With the patient prone on the examining table and the ankles clear of the table, the examiner squeezes the calf from side to side. Squeezing the calf deforms the soleus muscle and causes the overlying Achilles tendon to bow away from the tibia if the tendon is intact [88]. If there is plantar flexion of the foot, the test is negative and the Achilles tendon has not sustained a complete rupture. If plantar flexion is absent, the test indicates a total rupture.

The knee flexion test [89] also is performed in the prone position. The patient is asked to flex the knees to 90°. During inspection of this movement and when the tibia is vertical, the foot on the affected side falls into neutral or dorsiflexion (hyperdorsiflexion sign) and a rupture of the tendon is diagnosed [89].

Commonly, the tip-toe test is too painful in the acute situation, but is simple and effective in late and neglected ruptures; total rupture makes the patient unable to raise the heel off the ground on the injured side. Other tests described are the needle test [90], the sphygmomanometer test [91], and evaluation of plantar flexion strength.

In general, clinical examination is sufficient for a diagnosis of acute rupture of the Achilles tendon. More long-standing ruptures may produce ambiguous clinical findings and may need to be confirmed by imaging. Real time high-resolution ultrasonography and MRI provide an adjunct to clinical diagnosis. The reliability of the ultrasonography examination is investigator-dependent. Dynamic evaluation can be useful to determine whether the torn ends of the tendon are lying in close proximity to one another. The frayed tendon ends tend to overlap and might give the inexperienced ultrasonographer the false impression of an incomplete rupture.

Management

The goals of management of Achilles tendon ruptures are to minimize the morbidity of the injury, optimize rapid return to full function, and prevent complications. The variables that are evaluated most frequently in modern outcome studies after Achilles tendon rupture are complications to treatment, calf muscle strength, endurance, tendon configuration, patient satisfaction, and the impact of the Achilles tendon rupture on the absence from work and sports participation. Overall outcome measurements by 100-point scoring systems have been used [17,35,92,93]. A major limitation for their common use has been that the scores include dynamometry testing which is not widely available in routine clinical practice.

The complications can be divided into three categories: wound complications, general complications, and rerupture (Box 1). Further, complications can be rated as major or minor on the basis of their impact on activities of daily living. Deep venous thrombosis, pulmonary embolism, and rerupture are the most severe complications and may affect patients, regardless of treatment.

Several treatment methods and procedures have been described for the management of Achilles tendon rupture (Fig. 1). Despite the developments of the last decades, there is no consensus on the best way to deal with Achilles tendon ruptures. The modalities of management can be divided broadly into surgical and nonsurgical treatments. The surgical treatment methods can be

---

Box 1. Types of complications

Minor complications
Wound
    Superficial infection
    Wound hematoma
    Delayed wound healing
    Adhesion of the scar
    Suture granuloma
    Skin necrosis
General
    Pain
    Disturbance of sensibility
    Suture rupture
Major complications
Rerupture
Wound
    Deep infection
    Chronic fistula
General
    Marked tendon lengthening
    Pulmonary embolism
    Deep vein thrombosis
    Death

---

divided into open operative repair and percutaneous repair. In general, most surgeons suggest using operative management in physically active patients. Controversy exists about which surgical technique gives the best outcome.

Conservative management methods

The most common management protocol has been immobilization in a below-knee plaster cast in gravity equinus position for four weeks, and then placed into a more neutral position for a further four weeks [94–100]. In the British Isles, most orthopedic surgeons use a regime with a total of 6 weeks in a below-knee plaster cast. The gravity equinus position is maintained for 2 weeks, and then the foot is placed into a more neutral position for 2 more weeks. After this period, a change of plaster is performed; a below-knee plaster cast with the foot plantigrade is applied for an additional 2 weeks. Weight bearing is allowed for the last 2 weeks of this management regime. Some investigators have used an above-the-knee cast [101–104], but most patients find it cumbersome; the use of an above-the-knee cast probably is not warranted. Carden et al

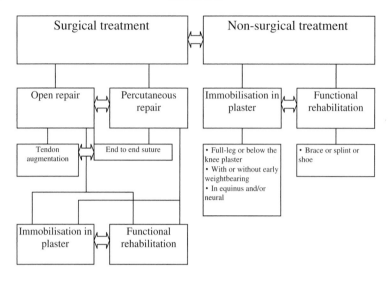

Fig. 1. Different methods of treatment of Achilles tendon rupture. Comparative studies between different treatment strategies are indicated with double arrows.

[44] found an increased risk for rerupture if nonsurgical management was not started within the first 48 hours following injury.

After 1 to 3 weeks of immobilization, braces, splints, or shoes with limitation of dorsiflexion and increased heel height have been used for functional rehabilitation [92,103,105,106]. The reports on early functional treatment suggest good functional outcome and low rerupture rates [3].

Surgical management

Open techniques

Many different open techniques of repair have been described, from end-to-end suturing to complex repairs with use of augmentation with fascial reinforcement or tendon grafts. The preferred method for early diagnosed ruptures has been simple end-to-end suture with Bunnell- or Kessler-type sutures placed 2 cm to 4 cm from the frayed tendon ends at the rupture site (Fig. 2). Because of the reported sural nerve injuries and wound complications (Fig. 3), many surgeons prefer a medial incision. End-to-end suturing can be performed under local anesthesia [107], and the tendon can be sutured through a 6 cm- to 8-cm long medial approach with low complication rates [108].

Augmentation is reserved commonly for late-presenting ruptures, neglected cases, or reruptures. When augmentation is performed, it usually is the second step of the operation and adds extra strength to the end-to-end suture. Local or distant tissue can be used to reinforce the tendon repair. Local tissue that is available for repair is the gastrocnemius fascia as a single turned-down strip [109,110]; as a single, rotated, and turned-down strip [111]; as two strips

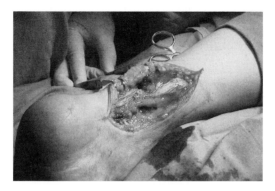

Fig. 2. A ruptured Achilles tendon at surgery. Note the horse tail appearance of the tendon ends, and the medial, curvilinear incision with an anterior apex, so that a wide flap lies over the Achilles tendon.

(one medial and one lateral) that are rotated and turned down [51]; or as a free flap [108]. Other local tissues that can be used for simple reinforcement or in a tendon transfer procedure are the plantaris tendon [112], the peroneus tendon [113], the flexor hallucis longus tendon [114], or the flexor digitorum longus tendon [115]. The distant tendons that are available are the fascia lata as a free flap [116] and the patellar–tendon–bone graft for reattachment of distal ruptures [117]. Artificial tendon implants, with materials, such as absorbable polymer-carbon fiber composites [118], knitted monofilament polypropylene [119], or collagen fiber prostheses [120], also have been used.

Percutaneous and minimally invasive techniques

Ma and Griffith [121] first described the percutaneous repair in 1977. Their method used six stab incisions: three lateral and three medial to the Achilles

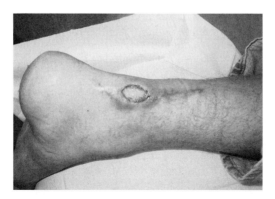

Fig. 3. Appearance of a superficial infection 6 weeks after open repair of a ruptured Achilles tendon in a 42-year-old recreational golfer who smoked 10 cigarettes per day. An end-to-end repair had been performed. The incision, although medial, lies directly over the tendon. We advocate a more medial, curvilinear incision with apex anterior so as to lift a wide flap over the Achilles tendon.

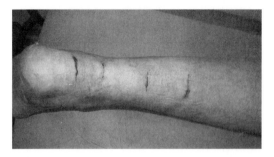

Fig. 4. Clinical appearance at 2 weeks following percutaneous repair of a ruptured Achilles tendon through four transverse incisions. Note the medial placement of the two most proximal transverse incisions to prevent injury to the sural nerve.

tendon. A suture is criss-crossed through the tendon and tied on the tendon surface. Many modifications of the percutaneous technique have been described [122–128]. Arthroscopy has been used as an adjunct to percutaneous techniques to allow direct visualization of the sural nerve and rupture site [126,129]; however, operating times increase and there is no evidence of improved clinical results.

We recently modified Webb and Bannister's [130] method of percutaneous surgery to produce a sound and secure repair which can be performed as an office procedure under local anesthesia (Fig. 4) [131]. In selected patients, we perform it through stab wounds, with no risk of injury to the sural nerve (Fig. 5). In the first 31 patients who were followed up for 3 years, no reruptures were experienced. Superficial wound problems, seen in 3 patients, were managed successfully with a short course of oral antibiotics.

A combined open and percutaneous operative technique has been devised for repair of Achilles tendon ruptures. Kakiuchi [132] and Assal et al [133] further developed the technique for limited open repair by the use of guided instrumentation. This procedure, with a 1.5-cm to 2-cm incision over the tendon

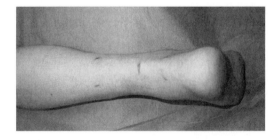

Fig. 5. Clinical appearance at 6 weeks following percutaneous repair of a ruptured Achilles tendon through five stab wounds in a 58-year-old female recreational tennis player. Note the transverse incision over the gap that was produced by the rupture of the tendon.

gap, allows the surgeon to visualize and control the tendon ends precisely while avoiding excessive dissection.

Overall, most studies demonstrated that the rate of rerupture is greater than that after open operative repair, because the repair usually is weaker than that achieved in open surgery. Also, there is an increased risk of sural nerve injury [1,134]. With the recent development of surgical techniques, percutaneous repair may be advocated in experienced hands as an alternative to open repair [126,128, 131,133,135–137].

Comparison of management strategies

Surgical versus nonsurgical management

The highest level of clinical evidence is derived from randomized, prospective studies; three such articles were published in the English language literature that compared the outcomes of surgical and nonsurgical treatment of Achilles tendon rupture [35,55,56]. Other randomized trials that were evaluated in the meta-analyses by Bhandari et al [8] and Khan et al [10] are derived from the German literature [136,139]. Further, the trials by Coombs [138] and Schroeder et al [139] were published as abstracts only.

Möller et al [35] performed a multi-center, prospective, randomized, controlled trail with 2 years of follow-up on 112 patients. The primary end point in the study was the rerupture rate. The study also included several methods of evaluation, including clinical examination, visual analog scores, functional performance testing, and time lost from work. Surgery consisted of a 6-cm to 8-cm long medial skin incision, an end-to-end suture without augmentation using a modified Kessler technique, and closure of the paratenon. The foot initially was placed in a below-knee plaster cast in equinus. At 12 days after surgery, the cast was replaced with an articulated brace that allowed a graduated increase in dorsiflexion over 8 weeks. Nonsurgical treatment consisted of immobilization in a below-knee plaster cast with the ankle in equinus for 4 weeks, followed by cast immobilization with the ankle in a neutral position for another 4 weeks. Both groups received a heel-raise of 15 mm for 4 to 8 weeks after removal of the cast or brace. More patients in the group that received nonsurgical treatment (11 of 53) sustained a rerupture than did those who underwent surgical treatment (1 in 59) ($P < .001$). Patients who had surgery reported a better quality of life during the 8-week treatment period ($P < .001$) and rated the result of treatment more highly ($P < .001$). Although there was no significant difference between the groups for length of time before return to work, patients with jobs that required mobility returned to work sooner after surgery ($P = .03$). Return to sports at 1 year, reduction in active plantar flexion, increased dorsiflexion, isokinetic strength, endurance testing, and the overall outcome score revealed no significant differences. The results following surgery may have resulted from the repair itself, the early functional rehabilitation, or a combination of both.

Cetti et al [56] found that open surgery with simple end-to-end sutures followed by cast immobilization resulted in a better outcome and patient satisfaction than nonsurgical treatment in a cast. The prospective, randomized trial included 111 patients, with a rerupture rate of 5.4% (3 in 56) after surgery and 12.7% (7 in 55) after nonsurgical treatment ($P = .19$). There was no significant difference in the mean length of time off work or major complications. Nonsurgical management resulted in lower rates of minor complications ($P = .004$). At 12 months of follow-up, the patients who had been managed surgically had a significantly greater rate of resuming sports activities at the same level, a lesser degree of calf atrophy, better ankle movement, and fewer complaints.

In 105 patients, nonsurgical management was favored because there were fewer complications [55], with rerupture rates of 4.5% in the surgical group and 8.0% in the nonsurgical group. The patients were evaluated clinically and with static and dynamic measurements of plantar flexion strength. Only minor, nonsignificant differences were noted between the final results in the two groups.

The meta-analysis by Bhandari et al [8] and the Cochrane review by Khan et al [10] identified and summarized the evidence from such trials on the effectiveness in the management of Achilles tendon ruptures. Further, systematic reviews of the literature of Achilles tendon rupture, including observational studies, have been presented using different methods to collect, include, and exclude data [3]. In general, however, there is an increased risk for rerupture following nonsurgical management and an increased risk for minor complications following surgical management.

The patient's attitudes must be taken into account, and a doctor–patient shared decision-making should consider outcome probabilities and patient preferences. Given the outcome probabilities and patient requirements, surgical management was the optimal strategy in an expected-value decision analysis [9]. For most patients, approximately twice as many reruptures can be prevented by surgery (approximately 10 out of 100 patients), with a risk of infection of approximately 5% [8]. Most infections can be treated successfully with antibiotics and do not necessitate a reoperation; the consequences of rerupture are considerably more serious.

Open repair versus percutaneous repair

Lim et al [140–143] performed a prospective, randomized, multi-center controlled trial with a minimum of 6 months follow-up in 66 patients to compare open and percutaneous repair of closed ruptured Achilles tendons. A modification of the technique that was described by Ma and Griffith [121] was used in the group that underwent percutaneous repair, whereas a Kessler suture that was supplemented with interrupted sutures was used in the group that underwent open surgery The complications in the group that had open repair (n = 33) included seven wound infections (21%), two adhesions (6%), and two reruptures (6%). In the group that had percutaneous repair (n = 33), 3 patients developed wound puckering (9%), 1 had a rerupture (3%), and 1 had persistent paresthesia in the sural nerve territory (3%). The difference in infective wound complications between the two groups was statistically significant ($P = .01$). The investigators advocated percutaneous repair on the basis of the low rate of complications and improved cosmetic appearance.

Majewski et al [137] compared the treatment of ruptured Achilles tendon by operative "end to end" surgery, percutaneous repair, or conservative therapy in 73 patients. After 2.5 years there were no differences; patients obtained an excellent or good result using a 100-point score. Patients in whom a percutaneous repair had been performed resumed work and sports activities sooner than the two other groups.

The systematic literature review by Wong et al [3] included 367 percutaneous repairs with a rerupture rate of 4.6%, wound complication rate of 6.5% (1.1% major), and a general complication rate of 11.4% (major 0.8%). The recent retrospective report by Halasi et al [126] of 144 percutaneous repairs from one center registered a rerupture rate of 4.2%, no wound or sural nerve complications, and a rate of general complications of 10.5% (partial rupture 2.8%, delayed healing 5.6%, deep vein thrombosis 2.1%).

Hockenbury and Johns [124] compared in vitro percutaneous repair [121] with open repair with the use of a Bunnell suture in transverse-sectioned Achilles tendons in 10 human cadavers. The tendons that were repaired with an open technique resisted almost twice as much ankle dorsiflexion before a 10 mm gap appeared in the repaired tendon. Modifications of the percutaneous Ma and Griffith [121] technique can improve the strength of the repair [144]. Also, it should be considered that in the original Ma and Griffith technique, a modified Bunnel monofilament suture was used, and the knot was tied outside of the tendon. More recently, we used multi-filament (eight strands) strong polytrimethylene carbonate (Maxon; Sherwood, Davis and Geck, St. Louis, Missouri) in a modified Kessler configuration, and the knot was tied within the substance of the tendon [131].

Percutaneous repair is associated with a shorter operation duration and lower risk of infection compared with open operative repair [10]. Overall, most studies on percutaneous repair demonstrated that the rate of repeat rupture is higher than after open operative repair [1,3], but are based on "older" percutaneous repair methods. More modern configurations have produced extremely low rerupture rates [135].

End-to-end suture versus tendon augmentation

Comparisons between simple end-to-end sutures and augmentation for the primary management of acute uncomplicated ruptures have been published, but no clinically significant differences have been detected [144–147]. Thus, primary augmentation of a repair of an acute rupture of the Achilles tendon is unwarranted, and a nonaugmented end-to-end repair is the management of choice

[7]. The strength of the repair differs according to the suture technique [148–151]. In a randomized trial, Mortensen et al [150] compared a weaker Mason suture technique with a stronger, reinforced continuous six-strand suture technique in end-to-end repair. The study included 57 patients who had an acute rupture of the Achilles tendon. Despite immobilization, separation developed after a biphasic course; after 7 weeks, the mean separation was 10.5 mm. No difference was found between the two techniques which suggested that there is no advantage to the more complicated suture techniques.

Postoperative treatment in a cast versus functional rehabilitation

The limits of desirable and undesirable stresses on the Achilles tendon during various phases of healing remains a challenge. Complete immobility without stress leads to tissue atrophy and adhesions, whereas too much stress too early is likely to jeopardize the tendon repair, lengthen the repair, or provoke a rerupture.

Many orthopedic surgeons in Europe have used the management protocol of surgical repair followed by below-knee cast immobilization [1]. Most investigators advocate a gradual reduction of gravity equinus to plantar flexion over 6 to 8 weeks.

During the last decades, many reports of good results following surgical repair and early motion or early weight bearing have been published [58,108,146, 149–171]. Functional rehabilitation may include the use of an orthosis, a splint, or a modified shoe. Many different functional rehabilitation protocols are advocated for 6 to 8 postoperative weeks, but it is difficult to compare and pool data from such studies. The functional rehabilitation regimens that are presented seem to be safe without an increase in the rerupture rate. Pooled data from five prospective comparative studies that investigated cast immobilization versus functional brace regimens [58,154,167,170,171] revealed a rerupture rate of 5.0% with cast immobilization and 2.3% with a functional brace ($P = .26$) [10]. Further, a postoperative functional brace seems to shorten the time needed for return to work and rehabilitation to sports [10].

We need to know much more about the optimal tendon strains and rehabilitation after an Achilles tendon injury. In an immobilized ankle, the addition of a 2.5-cm heel lift was sufficient to minimize plantar flexor activity during walking [169]. In one recent report, Arndt et al [170] measured the load on the Achilles tendon using an fiber optic technique in subjects who walked in a dynamic ankle foot orthosis that was set at positions used in standard rehabilitation protocols [58,108]. They related this loading to plantarflexor and dorsiflexor muscle activity. The dynamic orthosis limits ankle dorsiflexion but allows plantar flexion. The Achilles tendon force did not follow the intuitively expected pattern of greatest strain at the most dorsiflexed position. The lowest Achilles tendon force was recorded at $10°$ of plantar flexion, although no significant differences were found. These result indicate that other mechanisms besides the external, mechanical constraints that are placed by the dynamic ankle foot orthosis influence the load on the Achilles tendon [170].

Nonsurgical treatment: immobilization in plaster versus functional rehabilitation

Parallel with the increased use of postoperative functional treatment, functional nonsurgical management has gained increasing interest. In a randomized trial, Saleh et al [103] compared a dorsiflexion-limiting splint with immobilization in plaster. The functional treatment was appreciated by the patients, and mobility was restored more rapidly. Petersen et al [171] reported on 50 patients who had a first-time rupture of the Achilles tendon who were randomized to a cast or a CAM walker (BREG Inc., Vista, California). Both groups were treated for 8 weeks. They found five reruptures in 29 patients (17%) who were treated with a cast. No rerupture occurred in the 21 patients who were treated with a CAM walker. The difference was not statistically significant ($P = .07$). Given the possibility of type two error (44%), it is possible that a significant difference in the number of reruptures might have been noted if the number of patients had been larger.

Thermann et al [136] prospectively compared surgical and nonsurgical management with functional treatment with a boot (Variostabil, Frankfurt, Germany) in 50 patients (22 underwent operative treatment and 28 had conservative treatment). There were no significant differences in the functional results or in the course of healing. No rerupture was registered in either of the groups. Functional treatment in both groups allowed shorter periods of rehabilitation, and acceptance of the boot was particularly high in all patients. The same boot (Variostabil) was used in a prospective study of 161 patients in Braunschweig, Germany [172]. Nonsurgical functional boot management was indicated if dynamic ultrasonography showed sufficient adaptation of the rupture. Complications included seven cases of rerupture (4.3%). In the course of treatment, four patients (2.5%) suffered deep vein thrombosis of the leg; one case developed into postthrombotic syndrome.

Wallace et al [173] reported a series of 140 patients who were managed nonsurgically by a combined protocol that included the use of casts and a removable orthosis [106]. The overall complication rate was 8%, with three complete and five partial tendon reruptures, two deep vein thromboses, and one temporary dropfoot.

Other observational studies on nonsurgical functional management include small patient series. McComis et al [92] adapted the rehabilitation protocol that was developed by Carter et al [152] in the nonsurgical management of 15 patients; a functional brace allowed immediate weight bearing and active plantar flexion but limited dorsiflexion of the ankle with good results. Weber et al [174] treated 23 patients nonsurgically with an equinus ankle cast and boot. Major complications were reported in 6 of 23 patients; 4 experienced a rerupture 2 developed a deep vein thrombosis.

Limited conclusions can be drawn from the current literature on nonsurgical functional management [10].

Prognosis, return to sports, and patient-generated ratings of treatment

The time missed from work is highly dependent on the type of occupation. In heavy manual jobs, a period of sick leave of longer than 100 days can be expected. In sedentary work, a mean of about 30 days of sick leave has been reported. Möller et al [35] found a significant difference between patients who had light jobs and those who had heavy occupations, or were sedentary. Surgery and functional bracing produced 35 days of sick leave compared with nonsurgical management in a cast (67 days; $P = 0.03$).

Limping usually disappears after 12 to 14 weeks, and the triceps surae strength and endurance gradually improve during the first year [35]. The time to return to running or jumping sports usually is more than 6 months. Möller et al [35] found that 54% of the patients who had Achilles tendon rupture had resumed sports at the same level as before the injury, whereas approximately 30% had the ability but not the ambition to do so. Approximately 15% of the patients had not resumed sports at 1 year.

The impact of an Achilles tendon rupture is of greater importance than the management that is instituted [35,43,170]. Despite surgery, functional rehabilitation, and early weight bearing, residual strength deficit and muscle atrophy have not been prevented [35,170,171]. Deficits of plantar flexion in the range of 5% to 20% persist 1 year after the injury [35,170,175–182].

Summary

Achilles tendon ruptures are common, and their incidence is increasing. The evidence for best management is still controversial, and, in selected patients, conservative management and early mobilization achieves excellent results. Historically, surgery is associated with an increased risk of superficial skin breakdown; however, modern techniques of percutaneous repair that are performed under local anesthesia and are followed by early functional rehabilitation are becoming increasingly common, and should be considered. Appropriate randomized controlled trials are lacking (see Fig. 1); efforts should be made to run such studies to clarify the issues that were highlighted in this article.

References

[1] Maffulli N. Rupture of the Achilles tendon. J Bone Joint Surg Am 1999;81:1019–36.
[2] Maffulli N. The clinical diagnosis of subcutaneous tear of the Achilles tendon. A prospective study in 174 patients. Am J Sports Med 1998;26:266–70.
[3] Wong J, Barrass V, Maffulli N. Quantitative review of operative and nonoperative management of Achilles tendon ruptures. Am J Sports Med 2002;30:565–75.
[4] Wills CA, Washburn S, Caiozzo V, et al. Achilles tendon rupture. A review of the literature comparing surgical versus nonsurgical treatment. Clin Orthop 1986;207:156–63.
[5] Cetti R, Christensen SE, Ejsted R, et al. Operative versus nonoperative treatment of Achil-

les tendon rupture. A prospective randomized study and review of the literature. Am J Sports Med 1993;21(6):791–9.

[6] Lo IK, Kirkley A, Nonweiler B, et al. Operative versus nonoperative treatment of acute Achilles tendon ruptures: a quantitative review. Clin J Sport Med 1997;7(3):207–11.

[7] Popovic N, Lemaire R. Diagnosis and treatment of acute ruptures of the Achilles tendon. Current concepts review. Acta Orthop Belg 1999;65:458–71.

[8] Bhandari M, Guyatt GH, Siddiqui F, et al. Treatment of acute Achilles tendon ruptures: a systematic overview and metaanalysis. Clin Orthop 2002;400:190–200.

[9] Kocher MS, Bishop J, Marshall R, et al. Operative versus nonoperative management of acute Achilles tendon rupture: expected-value decision analysis. Am J Sports Med 2002; 30:783–90.

[10] Khan RK, Fick D, Brammar T, et al. Interventions for treating acute Achilles tendon ruptures. Cochrane Database Syst Rev 2004;3:CD003674.

[11] Cummins EJ, Anson BJ, Carr BW, et al. The structure of calcaneal tendon of Achilles in relation to orthopedic surgery. Surg Gynecol Obstet 1946;83:107–16.

[12] White JW. Torsion of the Achilles tendon; its surgical significance. Arch Surg 1943;46:784–7.

[13] Rufai A, Ralphs JR, Benjamin M. Structure and histopathology of the insertional region of the human Achilles tendon. J Orthop Res 1995;13:585–93.

[14] Elliot DH. Structure and function of mammalian tendon. Biol Rev Camb Philos Soc 1965; 40:392–421.

[15] Komi PV. Physiological and biomechanical correlates of muscle function: effects of muscle structure and stretch-shortening cycle on force and speed. Exerc Sport Sci Rev 1984;12: 81–121.

[16] Arndt AN, Komi PV, Brüggemann GP, et al. Individual muscle contributions to the in vivo Achilles tendon force. Clinical Biomechanics 1998;13:532–41.

[17] Thermann H, Frerichs O, Biewener A, et al. Biomechanical studies of human Achilles tendon rupture. Unfallchirurg 1995;98:570–5.

[18] Koivunen-Niemelä T, Parkkola K. Anatomy of the Achilles tendon (tendo calcaneus) with respect to tendon thickness measurements. Surg Radiol Anat 1995;17:263–8.

[19] Rosager S, Aagaard P, Dyhre-Poulsen P, et al. Load-displacement properties of the human triceps surae aponeurosis and tendon in runners and non-runners. Scand J Med Sci Sports 2002;12:90–8.

[20] Kallinen M, Suominen H. Ultrasonographic measurements of the Achilles tendon in elderly athletes and sedentary men. Acta Radiol 1994;35:560–3.

[21] Woo SL, Ritter MA, Amiel D, et al. The biomechanical and biochemical properties of swine tendons–long term effects of exercise on the digital extensors. Connect Tissue Res 1980;7: 177–83.

[22] Birch HL, McLaughlin L, Smith RK, et al. Treadmill exercise-induced tendon hypertrophy: assessment of tendons with different mechanical functions. Equine Vet J Suppl 1999; 30:222–6.

[23] Michna H. Morphometric analysis of loading-induced changes in collagen-fibril populations in young tendons. Cell Tissue Res 1984;236:465–70.

[24] Michna H. Tendon injuries induced by exercise and anabolic steroids in experimental mice. Int Orthop 1987;11:157–62.

[25] Shalabi A, Kristoffersen-Wiberg M, Aspelin P, et al. Immediate Achilles tendon adaptation following strength training of gastrocnemius-soleus complex evaluated by MRI. Med Sci Sports Exerc 2004;36:1841–6.

[26] Schatzker J, Brånemark PI. Intravital observations on the microvascular anatomy and microcirculation of the tendon. Acta Orthop Scand Suppl 1969;126:1–23.

[27] Barfred T. Achilles tendon rupture. Aetiology and pathogenesis of subcutaneous rupture assessed on the basis of the literature and rupture experiments on rats. Acta Orthop Scand Suppl 1973;3–126.

[28] Carr AJ, Norris SH. The blood supply of the calcaneal tendon. J Bone Joint Surg Br 1989; 71:100–1.

[29] Lagergren C, Lindholm A. Vascular distribution in the Achilles tendon; an angiographic and microangiographic study. Acta Chir Scand 1959;116:491–5.

[30] Stein V, Laprell H, Tinnemeyer S, et al. Quantitative assessment of intravascular volume of the human Achilles tendon. Acta Orthop Scand 2000;71:60–3.

[31] Reiter M, Ulreich N, Dirisamer A, et al. Colour and power Doppler sonography in symptomatic Achilles tendon disease. Int J Sports Med 2004;25:301–5.

[32] Hastad K, Larsson LG, Lindholm A. Clearance of radiosodium after local deposit in the Achilles tendon. Acta Chir Scand 1959;116:251–5.

[33] Aström M, Westlin N. Blood flow in the human Achilles tendon assessed by laser Doppler flowmetry. J Orthop Res 1994;12:246–52.

[34] Ohberg L, Lorentzon R, Alfredson H. Neovascularisation in Achilles tendons with painful tendinosis but not in normal tendons: an ultrasonographic investigation. Knee Surg Sports Traumatol Arthrosc 2001;9:233–8.

[35] Möller M, Movin T, Granhed H, et al. Acute rupture of tendon Achilles. A prospective randomised study of comparison between surgical and non-surgical treatment. J Bone Joint Surg Br 2001;83:843–8.

[36] Nillius SA, Nilsson BE, Westlin NE. The incidence of Achilles tendon rupture. Acta Orthop Scand 1976;47:118–21.

[37] Kannus P, Józsa L. Histopathological changes preceding spontaneous rupture of a tendon. A controlled study of 891 patients. J Bone Joint Surg Am 1991;73:1507–25.

[38] Möller A, Astron M, Westlin N. Increasing incidence of Achilles tendon rupture. Acta Orthop Scand 1996;67:479–81.

[39] Leppilahti J, Puranen J, Orava S. Incidence of Achilles tendon rupture. Acta Orthop Scand 1996;67:277–9.

[40] Levi N. The incidence of Achilles tendon rupture in Copenhagen. Injury 1997;28:311–3.

[41] Houshian S, Tscherning T, Riegels-Nielsen P. The epidemiology of Achilles tendon rupture in a Danish county. Injury 1998;29:651–4.

[42] Nyyssönen T, Lüthje P. Achilles tendon ruptures in South-East Finland between 1986–1996, with special reference to epidemiology, complications of surgery and hospital costs. Ann Chir Gynaecol 2000;89:53–7.

[43] Nestorson J, Movin T, Möller M, et al. Function after Achilles tendon rupture in the elderly: 25 patients older than 65 years followed for 3 years. Acta Orthop Scand 2000;71:64–8.

[44] Carden DG, Noble J, Chalmers J, et al. Rupture of the calcaneal tendon. The early and late management. J Bone Joint Surg Br 1987;69:416–20.

[45] Puddu G, Ippolito E, Postacchini F. A classification of Achilles tendon disease. Am J Sports Med 1976;4:145–50.

[46] Arndt KH. Achilles tendon rupture. Zentralbl Chir 1976;101:360–4.

[47] Jozsa L, Balint JB, Kannus P, et al. Distribution of blood groups in patients with tendon rupture. An analysis of 832 cases. J Bone Joint Surg Br 1989;71:272–4.

[48] Kujala UM, Järvinen M, Natri A, et al. ABO blood groups and musculoskeletal injuries. Injury 1992;23:131–3.

[49] Maffulli N, Reaper JA, Waterston SW, et al. ABO blood groups and Achilles tendon rupture in the Grampian Region of Scotland. Clin J Sport Med 2000;10:269–71.

[50] Davis JJ, Mason KT, Clark DA. Achilles tendon ruptures stratified by age, race, and cause of injury among active duty US military members. Mil Med 1999;164:872–3.

[51] Arner O, Lindholm A, Orell SR. Histologic changes in subcutaneous rupture of the Achilles tendon; a study of 74 cases. Acta Chir Scand 1959;116:484–90.

[52] Novacheck TF. Running injuries: a biomechanical approach. Instr Course Lect 1998;47: 397–406.

[53] Buchgraber A, Pässler HH. Percutaneous repair of Achilles tendon rupture. Immobilization versus functional postoperative treatment. Clin Orthop 1997;341:113–22.

[54] Winter E, Weise K, Weller S, et al. Surgical repair of Achilles tendon rupture. Comparison of surgical with conservative treatment. Arch Orthop Trauma Surg 1998;117:364–7.

[55] Nistor L. Surgical and non-surgical treatment of Achilles Tendon rupture. A prospective randomized study. J Bone Joint Surg Am 1981;63:394–9.

[56] Cetti R, Christensen SE, Ejsted R, et al. Operative versus nonoperative treatment of Achilles tendon rupture. A prospective randomized study and review of the literature. Am J Sports Med 1993;21:791–9.

[57] Fahlström M, Björnstig U, Lorentzon R. Acute Achilles tendon rupture in badminton players. Am J Sports Med 1998;26:467–70.

[58] Mortensen HM, Skov O, Jensen PE. Early motion of the ankle after operative treatment of a rupture of the Achilles tendon. A prospective, randomized clinical and radiographic study. J Bone Joint Surg Am 1999;81:983–90.

[59] Maffulli N, Ewen SW, Waterston SW, Reaper J, Barrass V. Tenocytes from ruptured and tendinopathic Achilles tendons produce greater quantities of type III collagen than tenocytes from normal Achilles tendons. An in vitro model of human tendon healing. Am J Sports Med 2000;28:499–505.

[60] Magnusson SP, Qvortrup K, Larsen JO, et al. Collagen fibril size and crimp morphology in ruptured and intact Achilles tendons. Matrix Biol 2002;21:369–77.

[61] Birk DE, Mayne R. Localization of collagen types I, III and V during tendon development. Changes in collagen types I and III are correlated with changes in fibril diameter. Eur J Cell Biol 1997;72:352–61.

[62] Corps AN, Robinson AH, Movin T, et al. Versican splice variant messenger RNA expression in normal human Achilles tendon and tendinopathies. Rheumatol 2004;43:969–72.

[63] Reed CC, Iozzo RV. The role of decorin in collagen fibrillogenesis and skin homeostasis. Glycoconj J 2002;19:249–55.

[64] Bernard-Beaubois K, Hecquet C, Hayem G, et al. In vitro study of cytotoxicity of quinolones on rabbit tenocytes. Cell Biol Toxicol 1998;14:283–92.

[65] Yoon JH, Brooks RL, Zhao JZ, et al. The effects of enrofloxacin on decorin and glycosaminoglycans in avian tendon cell cultures. Arch Toxicol 2004;78(10):599–608.

[66] Alfredson H, Pietilä T, Jonsson P, et al. Heavy-load eccentric calf muscle training for the treatment of chronic Achilles tendinosis. Am J Sports Med 1998;26:360–6.

[67] Nelen G, Martens M, Burssens A. Surgical treatment of chronic Achilles tendinitis. Am J Sports Med 1991;17:754–9.

[68] Coutts A, MacGregor A, Gibson J, et al. Clinical and functional results of open operative repair for Achilles tendon rupture in a nonspecialist surgical unit. J R Coll Surg Edinb 2002; 47(6):753–62.

[69] Cetti R, Junge J, Vyberg M. Spontaneous rupture of the Achilles tendon is preceded by widespread and bilateral tendon damage and ipsilateral inflammation: a clinical and histopathologic study of 60 patients. Acta Orthop Scand 2003;74:78–84.

[70] Bleakney RR, Tallon C, Wong JK, et al. Long-term ultrasonographic features of the Achilles tendon after rupture. Clin J Sport Med 2002;12:273–8.

[71] Orava S, Hurme M, Leppilahti J. Bilateral Achilles tendon rupture: a report on two cases. Scand J Med Sci Sports 1996;6:309–12.

[72] Kelly M, Dodds M, Huntley JS, et al. Bilateral concurrent rupture of the Achilles tendon in the absence of risk factors. Hosp Med 2004;65:310–1.

[73] Hayes T, McClelland D, Maffulli N. Metasynchronous bilateral Achilles tendon rupture. Bull Hosp Joint Dis 2003;61:140–4.

[74] Arøen A, Helgø D, Granlund OG, et al. Contralateral tendon rupture risk is increased in individuals with a previous Achilles tendon rupture. Scand J Med Sci Sports 2004;14:30–3.

[75] Fisher P. Role of steroids in tendon rupture or disintegration known for decades. Arch Intern Med 2004;164:678.

[76] Royer RJ, Pierfitte C, Netter P. Features of tendon disorders with fluoroquinolones. Therapie 1994;49:75–6.

[77] Vanek D, Saxena A, Boggs JM. Fluoroquinolone therapy and Achilles tendon rupture. J Am Podiatr Med Assoc 2003;93:333–5.

[78] Dodds WN, Burry HC. The relationship between Achilles tendon rupture and serum uric acid level. Injury 1984;16:94–5.

[79] Dent CM, Graham GP. Osteogenesis imperfecta and Achilles tendon rupture. Injury 1991;22: 239–40.

[80] Mathiak G, Wening JV, Mathiak M, et al. Serum cholesterol is elevated in patients with Achilles tendon ruptures. Arch Orthop Trauma Surg 1999;119:280–4.

[81] Ozgurtas T, Yildiz C, Serdar M, et al. Is high concentration of serum lipids a risk factor for Achilles tendon rupture? Clin Chim Acta 2003;331:25–8.

[82] von Bahr S, Movin T, Papadogiannakis N, et al. Mechanism of accumulation of cholesterol and cholestanol in tendons and the role of sterol 27-hydroxylase (CYP27A1). Arterioscler Thromb Vasc Biol 2002;22:1129–35.

[83] Inglis AE, Scott WN, Sculco TP, et al. Ruptures of the tendo achillis. An objective assessment of surgical and non-surgical treatment. J Bone Joint Surg Am 1976;58:990–3.

[84] Ballas MT, Tytko J, Mannarino F. Commonly missed orthopedic problems. Am Fam Physician 1998;57:267–74.

[85] Krueger-Franke M, Siebert CH, Scherzer S. Surgical treatment of ruptures of the Achilles tendon: a review of long-term results. Br J Sports Med 1995;29:121–5.

[86] Simmonds FA. The diagnosis of the ruptured Achilles tendon. Practitioner 1957;179:56–8.

[87] Thompson TC, Doherty JH. Spontaneous rupture of tendon of Achilles: a new clinical diagnostic test. J Trauma 1962;2:126–9.

[88] Scott BW, al Chalabi A. How the Simmonds-Thompson test works. J Bone Joint Surg Br 1992;74:314–5.

[89] Matles AL. Rupture of the tendo achilles: another diagnostic sign. Bull Hosp Joint Dis 1975; 36(1):48–51.

[90] O'Brien T. The needle test for complete rupture of the Achilles tendon. J Bone Joint Surg Am 1984;66:1099–101.

[91] Copeland SA. Rupture of the Achilles tendon: a new clinical test. Ann R Coll Surg Engl 1990;72:270–1.

[92] McComis GP, Nawoczenski DA, DeHaven KE. Functional bracing for rupture of the Achilles tendon. Clinical results and analysis of ground-reaction forces and temporal data. J Bone Joint Surg Am 1997;79:1799–808.

[93] Leppilahti J, Forsman K, Puranen J, et al. Outcome and prognostic factors of Achilles rupture repair using a new scoring method. Clin Orthop 1998;346:152–61.

[94] Edna TH. Non-operative treatment of Achilles tendon ruptures. Acta Orthop Scand 1980;51: 991–3.

[95] Gillies H, Chalmers J. The management of fresh ruptures of the tendo achillis. J Bone Joint Surg Am 1970;52:337–43.

[96] Jacobs D, Martens M, Van Audekercke R, et al. Comparison of conservative and operative treatment of Achilles tendon rupture. Am J Sports Med 1978;6:107–11.

[97] Lea RB, Smith L. Non-surgical treatment of tendo achillis rupture. J Bone Joint Surg Am 1972;54:1398–407.

[98] Lildholdt T, Munch-Jorgensen T. Conservative treatment to Achilles tendon rupture. A follow-up study of 14 cases. Acta Orthop Scand 1976;47:454–8.

[99] Nistor L. Conservative treatment of fresh subcutaneous rupture of the Achilles tendon. Acta Orthop Scand 1976;47:459–62.

[100] Persson A, Wredmark T. The treatment of total ruptures of the Achilles tendon by plaster immobilisation. Int Orthop 1979;3:149–52.

[101] Fruensgaard S, Helmig P, Riis J, et al. Conservative treatment for acute rupture of the Achilles tendon. Int Orthop 1992;16:33–5.

[102] Keller J, Rasmussen TB. Closed treatment of Achilles tendon rupture. Acta Orthop Scand 1984;55:548–50.

[103] Saleh M, Marshall PD, Senior R, et al. The Sheffield splint for controlled early mobilisation after rupture of the calcaneal tendon. A prospective, randomised comparison with plaster treatment. J Bone Joint Surg Br 1992;74:206–9.

[104] Stein SR, Luekens CA. Closed treatment of Achilles tendon ruptures. Orthop Clin N Am 1976;7:241–6.

[105] Thermann H, Hüfner T, Tscherne H. Achillessehnenruptur. [Achilles tendon rupture]. Orthopade [DE] 2000;29:235–50.

[106] Eames MH, Eames NW, McCarthy KR, et al. An audit of the combined non-operative and orthotic management of ruptured tendo Achillis. Injury 1997;28:289–92.

[107] Cetti R, Christensen SE. Surgical treatment under local anesthesia of Achilles tendon rupture. Clin Orthop 1983;173:204–8.

[108] Möller M, Karlsson J, Lind K, et al. Tissue expansion for repair of severely complicated Achilles tendon ruptures. Knee Surg Sports Traumatol Arthrosc 2001;9:228–32.

[109] Christensen R. To tilfaelde af subcutan Achillesseneruptur. [The management of subcutaneous rupture of the Achilles tendon]. Dansk Kir Sels Forh [DK] 1931;75:39.

[110] Bosworth DM. Repair of defects in the tendo achillis. J Bone Joint Surg Am 1956;38:111–4.

[111] Silfverskiöld N. Über die subutane totale Achillessehneruptur und deren Behandlung. [On subcutaneous rupture of the Achilles tendon and its management]. Acta Chir Scand [DE] 1941; 84:393–413.

[112] Lynn TA. Repair of the torn achilles tendon, using the plantaris tendon as a reinforcing membrane. J Bone Joint Surg Am 1966;48:268–72.

[113] Pérez Teuffer A. Traumatic rupture of the Achilles tendon. Reconstruction by transplant and graft using the lateral peroneus brevis. Orthop Clin N Am 1974;5:89–93.

[114] Wapner KL, Pavlock GS, Hecht PJ, et al. Repair of chronic Achilles tendon rupture with flexor hallucis longus tendon transfer. Foot Ankle 1993;14:443–9.

[115] Mann RA, Holmes GB, Seale KS, et al. Chronic rupture of the Achilles tendon: a new technique of repair. J Bone Joint Surg Am 1991;73:214–9.

[116] Zadek I. Repair of old rupture of tendo Achillis by means of fascia lata. J Bone Joint Surg Am 1940;22:1070–1.

[117] Besse JL, Lerat JL, Moyen B, et al. Reconstruction distale du tendon d'Achille avec un transplant ostendon à partir du système extenseur du genou. [Distal reconstruction of the Achilles tendon with a bone-tendon graft from extensor system of the knee]. Rev Chir Orthop Reparatrice Appar Mot [FR] 1995;81:453–7.

[118] Parsons JR, Rosario A, Weiss AB, et al. Achilles tendon repair with an absorbable polymer-carbon fiber composite. Foot Ankle 1984;5:49–53.

[119] Ozaki J, Fujiki J, Sugimoto K, et al. Reconstruction of neglected Achilles tendon rupture with Marlex mesh. Clin Orthop 1989;238:204–8.

[120] Kato YP, Dunn MG, Zawadsky JP, et al. Regeneration of Achilles tendon with a collagen tendon prosthesis. Results of a one-year implantation study. J Bone Joint Surg Am 1991;73:561–74.

[121] Ma GW, Griffith TG. Percutaneous repair of acute closed ruptured Achilles tendon: a new technique. Clin Orthop 1977;128:247–55.

[122] Rowley DI, Scotland TR. Rupture of the Achilles tendon treated by a simple operative procedure. Injury 1982;14:252–4.

[123] Klein W, Lang DM, Saleh M. The use of the Ma-Griffith technique for percutaneous repair of fresh ruptured tendo Achillis. Chir Organi Mov 1991;76:223–8.

[124] Hockenbury RT, Johns JC. A biomechanical in vitro comparison of open versus percutaneous repair of tendon Achilles. Foot Ankle 1990;11:67–72.

[125] FitzGibbons RE, Hefferon J, Hill J. Percutaneous Achilles tendon repair. Am J Sports Med 1993;21:724–7.

[126] Halasi T, Tállay A, Berkes I. Percutaneous Achilles tendon repair with and without endoscopic control. Knee Surg Sports Traumatol Arthrosc 2003;11:409–14.

[127] Gorschewsky O, Pitzl M, Pütz A, et al. Percutaneous repair of acute Achilles tendon rupture. Foot Ankle Int 2004;25:219–24.

[128] Haji A, Sahai A, Symes A, et al. Percutaneous versus open tendo achillis repair. Foot Ankle Int 2004;25:215–8.

[129] Thermann H, Tibesku CO, Mastrokalos DS, et al. Endoscopically assisted percutaneous Achilles tendon suture. Foot Ankle Int 2001;22:158–60.

[130] Webb JM, Bannister GC. Percutaneous repair of the ruptured tendo Achillis. J Bone Joint Surg Br 1999;81:877–80.
[131] McClelland D, Maffulli N. Percutaneous repair of ruptured Achilles tendon. J R Coll Surg Edinb 2002;47:613–8.
[132] Kakiuchi M. A combined open and percutaneous technique for repair of tendo Achillis. Comparison with open repair. J Bone Joint Surg Br 1995;77:60–3.
[133] Assal M, Jung M, Stern R, et al. Limited open repair of Achilles tendon ruptures: a technique with a new instrument and findings of a prospective multicenter study. J Bone Joint Surg Am 2002;84-A:161–70.
[134] Aracil J, Pina A, Lozano JA, et al. Percutaneous suture of Achilles tendon ruptures. Foot Ankle 1992;13:350–1.
[135] Cretnik A, Kosanovic M, Smrkolj V. Percutaneous suturing of the ruptured Achilles tendon under local anesthesia. J Foot Ankle Surg 2004;43:72–81.
[136] Thermann H, Zwipp H, Tscherne H. Die funcktionelle Behandlung der frischen Achillessehnrupture. 2 Jahre Ergebnisse von einem voraussichtlichen randomisierten Studium. [Functional treatment concept of acute rupture of the Achilles tendon. 2 years results of a prospective randomized study]. Unfallchirurg [DE] 1995;98:21–32.
[137] Majewski M, Rickert M, Steinbrück K. Achilles tendon rupture. A prospective study assessing various treatment possibilities. Orthopade 2000;29:670–6.
[138] Coombs RRH. Prospective trial of conservative and surgical treatment of Achilles tendon rupture [abstract]. J Bone Joint Surg Br 1981;63:288.
[139] Schroeder D, Lehmann M, Steinbruck K. Treatment of acute achilles tendon ruptures: open vs. percutaneous repair vs. conservative treatment. A prospective randomized study. Orthopaedic Transactions 1997;21:1228.
[140] Lim J, Dalal R, Waseem M. Percutaneous vs. open repair of the ruptured Achilles tendon—a prospective randomized controlled study. Foot Ankle Int 2001;22:559–68.
[141] Cretnik A, Zlajpah L, Smrkolj V, et al. The strength of percutaneous methods of repair of the Achilles tendon: a biomechanical study. Med Sci Sports Exerc 2000;32:16–20.
[142] Jessing P, Hansen E. Surgical treatment of 102 tendo achillis ruptures—suture or tenontoplasty? Acta Chir Scand 1975;141:370–7.
[143] Rantanen J, Hurme T, Paananen M. Immobilization in neutral versus equinus position after Achilles tendon repair. A review of 32 patients. Acta Orthop Scand 1993;64:333–5.
[144] Nyyssönen T, Saarikoski H, Kaukonen JP, et al. Simple end-to-end suture versus augmented repair in acute Achilles tendon ruptures: a retrospective comparison in 98 patients. Acta Orthop Scand 2003;74:206–8.
[145] Beskin JL, Sanders RA, Hunter SC, et al. Surgical repair of Achilles tendon ruptures. Am J Sports Med 1987;15:1–8.
[146] Cetti R. Ruptured Achilles tendon—preliminary results of a new treatment. Br J Sports Med 1988;22:6–8.
[147] Krackow KA, Thomas SC, Jones LC. A new stitch for ligament-tendon fixation. Brief note. J Bone Joint Surg Am 1986;68:764–6.
[148] Mortensen NH, Saether J. Achilles tendon repair: a new method of Achilles tendon repair tested on cadaverous materials. J Trauma 1991;31:381–4.
[149] Mortensen NH, Saether J, Steinke MS, et al. Separation of tendon ends after Achilles tendon repair: a prospective, randomized, multicenter study. Orthopedics 1992;15:899–903.
[150] Marti R, Weber BG. Rupture of the Achilles tendon—functional after care. Helv Chir Acta 1974;41:293–6.
[151] Cetti R, Henriksen LO, Jacobsen KS. A new treatment of ruptured Achilles tendons. A prospective randomized study. Clin Orthop 1994;308:155–65.
[152] Carter TR, Fowler PJ, Blokker C. Functional postoperative treatment of Achilles tendon repair. Am J Sports Med 1992;20:459–62.
[153] Armbrecht A, Zenker W, Egbers HJ, et al. Plaster-free, early functional after-care of surgically managed Achilles tendon rupture. Chirurg 1993;64(11):926–30.

[154] Saw Y, Baltzopoulos V, Lim A, et al. Early mobilization after operative repair of ruptured Achilles tendon. Injury 1993;24(7):479–84.

[155] Solveborn SA, Moberg A. Immediate free ankle motion after surgical repair of acute Achilles tendon ruptures. Am J Sports Med 1994;22:607–10.

[156] Troop RL, Losse GM, Lane JG, et al. Early motion after repair of Achilles tendon ruptures. Foot Ankle Int 1995;16:705–9.

[157] Mandelbaum BR, Myerson MS, Forster R. Achilles tendon ruptures. A new method of repair, early range of motion, and functional rehabilitation. Am J Sports Med 1995;23:392–5.

[158] Fernández-Fairén M, Gimeno C. Augmented repair of Achilles tendon ruptures. Am J Sports Med 1997;25:177–81.

[159] Motta P, Errichiello C, Pontini I. Achilles tendon rupture. A new technique for easy surgical repair and immediate movement of the ankle and foot. Am J Sports Med 1997;25:172–6.

[160] Aoki M, Ogiwara N, Ohta T, et al. Early active motion and weightbearing after cross-stitch achilles tendon repair. Am J Sports Med 1998;26:794–800.

[161] Robinson PS, Lin TW, Reynolds PR, et al. Strain-rate sensitive mechanical properties of tendon fascicles from mice with genetically engineered alterations in collagen and decorin. J Biomech Eng 2004;126:252–7.

[162] Speck M, Klaue K. Early full weightbearing and functional treatment after surgical repair of acute Achilles tendon rupture. Am J Sports Med 1998;26:789–93.

[163] Roberts CP, Palmer S, Vince A, et al. Dynamised cast management of Achilles tendon ruptures. Injury 2001;32:423–6.

[164] Kerkhoffs GM, Struijs PA, Raaymakers EL, et al. Functional treatment after surgical repair of acute Achilles tendon rupture: wrap vs walking cast. Arch Orthop Trauma Surg 2002;122: 102–5.

[165] Costa ML, Shepstone L, Darrah C, et al. Immediate full-weight-bearing mobilisation for repaired Achilles tendon ruptures: a pilot study. Injury 2003;34:874–6.

[166] Rolf C, Movin T. Etiology, histopathology, and outcome of surgery in achillodynia. Foot Ankle Int 1997;18:565–9.

[167] Kangas J, Pajala A, Siira P, et al. Early functional treatment versus early immobilization in tension of the musculotendinous unit after Achilles rupture repair: a prospective, randomized, clinical study. J Trauma 2003;54:1171–80 [discussion 11: 1180–1].

[168] Maffulli N, Tallon C, Wong J, Lim KP, Bleakney R. Early weightbearing and ankle mobilization after open repair of acute midsubstance tears of the Achilles tendon. Am J Sports Med 2003;31:692–700.

[169] Akizuki KH, Gartman EJ, Nisonson B, et al. The relative stress on the Achilles tendon during ambulation in an ankle immobiliser: implications for rehabilitation after Achilles tendon repair. Br J Sports Med 2001;35:329–33.

[170] Arndt A, Ryberg Å, Komi P, et al. Efficacy of ankle foot orthoses in unloading the Achilles tendon and the effect of muscle activity. Presented at the Orthopaedic Research Society Meeting. 2005.

[171] Petersen OF, Nielsen MB, Jensen KH, et al. Randomized comparison of CAM walker and light-weight plaster cast in the treatment of first-time Achilles tendon rupture. Ugeskr Laeger 2002;164:3852–5.

[172] Reilmann H, Förster EW, Weinberg AM, et al. Konservative praktische Therapie geschlossenen von der Achillessehne. Behandlungsannäherung und Analyse der Ergebnisse. [Conservative functional therapy of closed rupture of the Achilles tendon. Treatment approach and analysis of results.] Unfallchirurg [DE] 1996;99:576–80.

[173] Wallace RG, Traynor IE, Kernohan WG, et al. Combined conservative and orthotic management of acute ruptures of the Achilles tendon. J Bone Joint Surg Am 2004;86-A: 1198–202.

[174] Weber M, Niemann M, Lanz R, et al. Nonoperative treatment of acute rupture of the Achilles tendon: results of a new protocol and comparison with operative treatment. Am J Sports Med 2003;31:685–91.

[175] Arner O, Lindholm A. Subcutaneous rupture of the Achilles tendon; a study of 92 cases. Acta Chir Scand 1959;116:1–51.

[176] Leppilahti J, Puranen J, Orava S. ABO blood group and Achilles tendon rupture. Ann Chir Gynaecol 1996;85:369–71.

[177] Maffulli N, Barrass V, Ewen SW. Light microscopic histology of Achilles tendon ruptures. A comparison with unruptured tendons. Am J Sports Med 2000;28:857–63.

[178] Maffulli N, Waterston SW, Squair J, et al. Changing incidence of Achilles tendon rupture in Scotland: a 15-year study. Clin J Sport Med 1999;9:157–60.

[179] Marti R, Weber BG. Abbruch von der Achillessehne. Praktisch nach Sorge. [Rupture of the achilles tendon - functional after care]. Helv Chir Acta [DE] 1974;41:293–6.

[180] Möller M, Lind K, Movin T, et al. Calf muscle function after Achilles tendon rupture. A prospective, randomised study comparing surgical and non-surgical treatment. Scand J Med Sci Sports 2002;12:9–16.

[181] Matles AL. Rupture of the tendo achilles: another diagnostic sign. Bull Hosp Joint Dis 1975;36:48–51.

[182] Zantop T, Tillmann B, Petersen W. Quantitative assessment of blood vessels of the human Achilles tendon: an immunohistochemical cadaver study. Arch Orthop Trauma Surg 2003; 123:501–4.

ELSEVIER
SAUNDERS

Foot Ankle Clin N Am
10 (2005) 357–370

FOOT AND
ANKLE CLINICS

Neglected Ruptures of the Achilles Tendon

Hamish D.H. Leslie, MB, ChB, FRACS,
W.H.B. Edwards, MB, BS, Dip Anat, MS,
FRACS (Orth), FAOrthA*

*Orthopaedic Foot and Ankle Centre of Victoria, Level 1, Victoria House, 316-324 Malvern Road,
Prahran, Victoria, 3181 Australia*

Hippocrates wrote of the Achilles tendon, "this tendon, if bruised or cut, causes the most acute fevers, induces choking, deranges the mind and at length brings death." Although the prognosis of this injury has improved, the management remains controversial. The role of operative and nonoperative treatment of acute ruptures continues to be debated [1–7], but most investigators agree that neglected ruptures should be treated operatively unless there are significant contraindications to surgery or the patient has minimal functional demands. A wide variety of management options is available.

The definition of an old, chronic, or neglected rupture is variable. The most commonly used timeframe, which also is used in this article, is 4 weeks from the time of injury [8–13]. Similarly, when there has been a delay in treatment, ruptures may be called chronic [11,14–17], neglected [10,18–25] or old [26,27].

This article reviews the pathophysiology, triceps surae function, patient evaluation and focuses on the management of neglected ruptures of the Achilles tendon.

Pathology/pathophysiology

In 1931, Platt [28] wrote "in untreated ruptures the thickened sheath becomes adherent to the tendon ends and acts a feeble bond of union... the power of plantar flexion is permanently impaired."

---

* Corresponding author.

E-mail address: willedwards@vicfoot.com (W.H.B. Edwards).

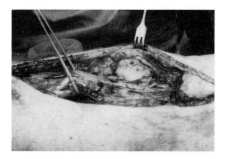

Fig. 1. An operative specimen where the proximal stump (held in loop) is adherent to the fascia posterior to the flexor hallucis longus.

This is a similar finding to Zadek [26]; Zadek [27] found no tendinous tissue inside the sheath at the site of the defect, a conical-shaped proximal tendon stump, and a bulbous distal stump. The proximal tendon stump is often adherent to the posterior fascia of the flexor hallucis longus (Fig. 1). The tendon of plantaris, if present, may be hypertrophied. Another common finding is thick scar tissue that bridges the site of rupture (Fig. 2) [7,12,21,29], because partial regeneration of the calcaneal tendon may occur, at least in animals [30]. By 56 days following calcaneal tendon resection in rabbits, a well-organized connective tissue was formed, although by 240 days it never displayed the fascicular arrangement of tendon. This tissue is not as strong as normal tendon, and hence, elongates with time [7,31]. Whatever the pathologic findings at the site of rupture, there usually is a gap between the tendon ends, with retraction of the proximal stump that results in shortening of the triceps surae muscle bellies, and hence, weakness of plantar flexion of the ankle. The tension that the muscle fiber can produce decreases as the fiber shortens, until it becomes zero when the fiber is approximately 60% of its resting length [32].

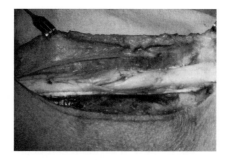

Fig. 2. Achilles tendon in continuity but with grossly abnormal tissue bridging the gap between the proximal and distal ends.

Triceps surae function

There has been disagreement about the functional importance of the triceps surae during gait. Boyd [33] performed a complete transverse tenotomy of the Achilles tendon on 24 patients for intermittent claudication. Although plantar flexion was weakened, gait was "almost normal" and "most patients are able to rise on their toes." More recent gait analysis studies showed a more profound disturbance of gait. Sutherland et al [34] and Simon et al [35] studied patients who had amputation and neuromuscular deficit, normal subjects, and subjects following tibial nerve block. Sutherland et al [34] found that the ankle plantar flexors contributed to knee and ankle stability, restrained forward rotation of the tibia on the talus, and conserved energy by minimizing vertical oscillation of the body's center of mass. Simon et al [35] concluded that calf muscle activity is used to restrain the body's forward momentum rather than to propel it forward. As Sutherland et al [34] noted, however, tibial nerve block anesthetizes the sole of the foot and paralyzes the whole of the posterior calf musculature, and, therefore, does not produce a true picture of isolated triceps surae dysfunction.

Murray et al [36] studied the gait of a woman who had her triceps surae excised for sarcoma. They found that she had a "mild disability" with regard to gait and retained 38% of her normal plantar flexion strength. She could not, however, increase walking speed beyond normal, run, or stand on tiptoes. Barnes and Hardy's [12] paper included gait analysis of two patients who refused operative reconstruction of a neglected rupture. Both walked with a marked limp, were unable to run, stand on tiptoes or play sports, and climbed stairs flatfooted. They demonstrated weakness similar to that found by Murray et al [36] but, due to fatigue, the investigators were unable to obtain endurance figures.

Diagnosis and patient evaluation

Treatment delay is secondary to late patient presentation or initial misdiagnosis. There often is a history of insignificant trauma; the patient can still walk and plantarflex the ankle, and there may be no palpable tendon gap. Older series [5,9,29] reported initial misdiagnosis rates of 18% to 27%.

Patients who have a neglected rupture often recall a traumatic event and may present because of a disability, such as limp, ankle swelling, or inability to run or climb stairs. Functional limitation should be assessed as well as anesthetic and surgical risk factors, including smoking, peripheral vascular disease, and deep vein thrombosis. On presentation, limp, ankle swelling, and increased dorsiflexion of the ankle often are present. Calf wasting and a palpable gap (Fig. 3) may be present. Triceps surae strength can be established by observing normal and tiptoe gait, and by the double- and single-leg heel-rise test. Some patients can perform a single heel rise but generally cannot do so repetitively [7].

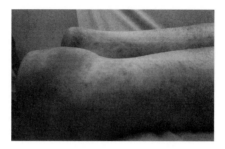

Fig. 3. Clinical example of a visible (and palpable) gap.

Thompson's [37] calf squeeze test often helps to confirm the diagnosis but is not always reliable in a neglected rupture [12]. The status of the skin and vascularity of the limb also should be assessed.

The size of the gap should be documented because this will help to guide surgical management [7]. Ultrasonography and MRI (Fig. 4) can help to confirm diagnosis and document the extent of the tendon gap. At ultrasonography, the normal tendon is a hypoechogenic band with well-defined echogenic margins. Complete tears display tendon discontinuity and decreased and increased echogenicity, depending on the chronicity of the injury [6,38]. On MRI, the tendon is seen as an area of low signal intensity of all pulse sequences [6]. In the axial plane, a normal tendon appears crescentic and both limbs can be compared. The sagittal plane shows the extent of the tear best.

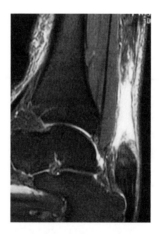

Fig. 4. Sagittal plane MRI of a chronic rupture.

Complete tears show discontinuity and altered signal on T2-weighted scans [6,39].

Management

Nonoperative

In 1953, Christensen [42] reported what may have been the largest series of neglected ruptures that were treated conservatively. Eighteen of 51 patients who had 57 ruptures (nearly two thirds of which were neglected) were treated conservatively because the operation was contraindicated, they refused surgery, of the 18 patients treated conservatively had ruptures several months old and were showing signs of regaining strength and hence the injury was managed "expectantly" (11 patients). "Satisfactory" results (ie, normal gait, return to previous occupation, and slight or no discomfort) were obtained in 75% of patients who underwent surgery and 56% of patients who were managed conservatively. In addition, improvement in all patients who did not undergo surgery occurred slowly, sometimes over several years. Brace management should be considered in patients who do not have a functional deficit, and in those who have potential wound healing problems or anesthetic contraindications to surgery. An ankle foot orthosis, with or without ankle hinge, may be used [7].

Operative

Patients who have a neglected rupture and a functional deficit are managed optimally with surgery [5,7,10,18,41] with direct tendon apposition (Fig. 5) [7,10]. Surgery should aim to achieve tendon continuity with a robust repair and tension equal to that of the opposite limb. Following debridement of the tendon ends and with retraction of the proximal tendon fragment, however, a large gap may be present. Although intraoperative traction of the proximal tendon using a weight may close this gap [7], often this is not possible, and hence, routine tendon repair techniques cannot be used. This, in part, explains the large variety of operative techniques that is described for this condition.

There is some debate regarding whether delayed surgical management impairs the functional result. Boyden et al [13] compared 11 patients who received late reconstruction (4 or more weeks following injury) with 10 patients who received early reconstruction (within 1 week of injury). Both groups had end-to-end repair—usually with augmentation (plantaris or Achilles turndown flap)—with assessments at least 4 years postoperatively. Follow-up included subjective (pain, functional/recreational limitation, satisfaction, appearance) and objective (physical examination, instrumented strength testing, gait analysis) assessment. The two groups were comparable, although only 8 of the patients who had late reconstruction and 7 of the patients who had early reconstruction

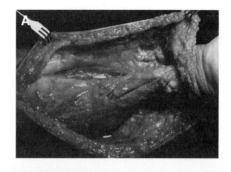

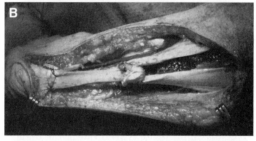

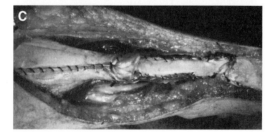

Fig. 5. (*A*) Operative example of direct repair and shortening of chronic rupture. (*B*) Clinical example of an Achilles tendon turndown in preparation. (*C*) Same patient with completed turndown.

were available for objective assessment. Inglis and Sculco [2] compared 34 patients who had early repair (within 1 month of injury) with 16 patients who had late repair (1 month or later); although strength and power measurements were comparable, the group that had late repair had a 20% reduction of endurance. They also found greater calf atrophy in the patients who had late repair, but this did not correlate with power or strength measurements or functional results. Christensen [40] compared 10 "early" repairs (average 35 days from injury to repair) with 10 "late" repairs (average 390 days from injury to repair) and, using the above outcome criteria, the results were "equally good".

The techniques for repair or reconstruction of the neglected rupture can be classified broadly as end-to-end repair, tendo-Achilles advancement or flap reconstruction, local tendon transfer, and implantation (autograft, allograft, or synthetic).

Tendo-Achilles advancement or flap reconstruction

Tendo-Achilles advancement can allow end-to-end apposition of ruptured tendon ends that are separated by a large gap. In 1975, Abraham and Pankovich [23] described this technique in four patients. An inverted "V" incision was made at the musculotendinous junction; the arms of the "V" were at least 1.5 times the length of the tendon defect to allow suturing of the incision in a "Y" configuration. Gaps up to 6 cm could be closed with this technique. Three patients gained full strength of the triceps surae and one had slight weakness. The only complication was one sural nerve neuroma. Leitner et al [27] reported on three patients who had tendon defects of 9 cm to 10 cm who were managed successfully using this technique. Kissel et al [42] used the same technique, augmented with a plantaris weave and pull-out suture in 14 patients. Parker and Repinecz [22] described a similar technique in which a tongue-in-groove advancement of the gastrocnemius aponeurosis was used to close a 6.5-cm defect in one patient. Compared to V-Y advancement, they reported this technique to be easier to perform and more length can be accomplished, 50% more, if necessary.

Several different turndown flaps of the Achilles tendon have been recommended to bridge the tendon gap or to augment another method of repair. Christensen, in 1931, first described this technique and later reported on 35 acute and neglected tears [40]. A distally based 2 cm by 10 cm flap was cut in the proximal tendon fragment, turned down to cover the tendon defect or previous repair, and the defect that was created by the flap was closed (Fig. 5). Postoperatively, the patient was in an equinus above-knee plaster for 5 weeks. A walking below-knee cast was applied for another 5 weeks. Two reruptures occurred and 75% of outcomes were classified as "satisfactory." Arner and Lindholm [29] reported 86 operatively treated acute and neglected cases. Twenty had simple end-to-end repair, but 66 received supplementation of this repair with three different techniques: Christensen's (n = 30); Silfverskiold's (similar to Christensen but the graft was rotated through 180°, hence the smooth surface faced posteriorly; n =25); and the remainder with their own technique, similar to Silfverskiold's, but instead two flaps (one medial and one lateral) are rotated. The functional results of these four techniques were "approximately equal," but their technique produced less tethering of the scar. Gerdes et al [43] described a modified Lindholm technique [29] that was used in seven patients, only one of which was a chronic rupture. Their cadaver study showed that flap augmentation repair had a 41% greater ultimate tensile strength than simple suture repair alone. They also allowed immediate postoperative weight bearing in a below-knee cast, with cast removal at 6 weeks.

In Rush's [21] technique, the flap was tubularized, and all five patients who had neglected ruptures "were happy with the result." Bosworth [31] reported on seven patients, five of whom had neglected ruptures that were repaired with a 0.5-inch wide strip of the proximal aponeurosis that was woven through the proximal and distal tendon stumps. No complications occurred. Other investigators have used V-Y advancement and flap turndown in combination [24] or as isolated techniques [12] with good results.

Local tendon transfer

The use of the plantaris tendon, if present, may be regarded as a tendon transfer or local tissue augmentation of a repair. Its use in Achilles tendon repair was described first by Gilcreest [44] who sutured the repair with the plantaris tendon—leaving it attached distally—and reinforced the repair with fascia lata strips. Lynn [45] detached the plantaris from its insertion and fanned it out to reinforce end-to-end Achilles repair in 18 patients. These were acute ruptures, however, and he emphasized that this technique could not be used in neglected ruptures because the plantaris becomes incorporated in the "cicatricial mass," Schedl and Fasol [46] compared the results of repair with the plantaris tendon (divided at the musculo–tendon junction, woven through proximal and distal stumps, then fanned out over the repair) with direct repair with 3/0 polyglycol suture. The only difference was that the group in which polyglycol suture was used convalesced more quickly and the fanned plantaris seemed to help avoid painful scar adhesion. Only 2 of the 56 patients, however, had neglected ruptures. Other studies have used the plantaris as one of several techniques of primary repair [47,48] or to augment another technique of repair [13,18,28,].

Platt [28], in 1931, was the first to describe a "true" local tendon transfer to repair a neglected rupture when he, among other techniques, transferred the peroneus longus and tibialis posterior to the calcaneus. Since then, the peroneus brevis [8,17,48–50], flexor digitorum longus (FDL) [14], and flexor hallucis longus (FHL) [14,18,51,52] have been used.

White and Kraynick [49] first reported a neglected rupture that was reconstructed with a peroneus brevis transfer to the calcaneus and reinforced with fascial strips. Teuffer [50] described passing the peroneus brevis tendon through the calcaneus, across the repair site, and suturing it to the proximal Achilles tendon. All 30 of his patients had good or excellent results, but he did not mention using this technique for a neglected rupture. Turco and Spinella [17] augmented end-to-end repair of the Achilles tendon with a modification of Teuffer's technique, by passing the peroneus brevis through the distal tendon stump, rather than the calcaneus. Weight bearing was commenced in a below-knee cast 2 weeks postoperatively, with cast removal at 6 to 8 weeks. This series involved 40 patients and included 24 neglected ruptures and 4 reruptures. Although excellent results were reported, the criteria by which these results were obtained was not identified. Two concerns, however, have been raised about this technique. First, the potential for eversion weakness [7,14,52]. St. Pierre et al [53], however, showed no significant loss of eversion strength following Evan's lateral ligament reconstruction. This may be because the peroneus longus has more than twice the strength of eversion of the peroneus brevis [54]. Secondly, because the tendon was placed distally in a lateral to medial direction, it does not duplicate the medial pull of the normal Achilles tendon [14].

Mann et al [14] used the FDL to bridge the gap in seven chronic tendo-Achilles ruptures. The FDL tendon was harvested in the midfoot, and the distal stump was sutured to the FHL. They also included a proximal fascial turndown flap in all cases and, when length allowed, the proximal stump was reattached to the calcaneus with a pull-out wire technique. Postoperatively, an equinus nonweight-bearing cast was applied for 4 weeks, followed by a weight-bearing cast for another 4 weeks, and then a removable brace for 3 months. They had six good or excellent results, no reruptures, and no functional disability secondary to loss of the FDL.

Hansen [51] described the use of the FHL, harvested through an incision in the anterior paratenon of the Achilles tendon, to augment a proximal tendon flap or free fascial graft that was used to bridge a defect in a delayed rupture. He advocated that the FHL muscle belly augmented the strength of the triceps surae and also improved the tendon's blood supply. Wapner et al [18] reported on eight neglected ruptures that were reconstructed with the FHL transfer that was harvested from the midfoot (Fig. 6). Once harvested, the tendon was passed through a drill hole in the calcaneus, then woven through the Achilles tendon. Three cases were supplemented with a plantaris weave or proximal Achilles tendon turndown. Results were available for seven patients, six of whom obtained good or excellent results according to Mann et al's [14] criteria. Cybex testing revealed a 29.5% decrease in plantar flexion power compared with the nonoperated ankle. No functional disability was noted secondary to the FHL harvest. This is in agreement with Frenette and Jackson [55] who reported 10 cases of FHL tendon laceration in young athletes, four of which were not repaired, with no disability evident. Wapner et al [18] believed that the theoretic advantages of the FHL transfer include a long durable tendon with a stronger muscle than other tendon transfers; the axis of FHL contraction most closely reproduces the Achilles tendon; FHL fire in phase with triceps surae; anatomic proximity makes harvesting easy; maintenance of normal muscle balance of the ankle (ie, plantar flexor to plantar flexor); and that their technique adds 10 cm to 12 cm of tendon compared with Hansen's technique, which allows weaving of the tendon through the Achilles. This technique is similar to that used by Myerson [7]; Wilcox et al [15], who treated 20 patients who had chronic Achilles

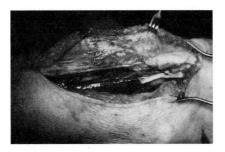

Fig. 6. Flexor hallucis longus transfer to the os calcis with the Achilles tendon excised.

tendinopathy; and Dalal and Zenios [16], who reported excellent results following reconstruction of three chronic ruptures in two elderly patients.

Implantation

Implantation of material may be used to augment a repair or bridge a gap in a neglected rupture. Materials that have been used previously include autograft, allograft, and synthetic material.

Autografts.   Platt [28] described three patients who had reinforcement of end-to-end repair of neglected ruptures with fascia lata and one in which a large gap was bridged with a semitendinosus free tendon graft. Zadek [27] used three strips of fascia lata to bridge a 3-inch gap in a neglected rupture with a good result. Tobin [19] treated seven patients who had a neglected ruptured or severed Achilles tendons (six were more than 4 weeks following injury), with a "tube" of fascia lata. The results were "uniformly good." Bugg and Boyd [20] reported treating 21 Achilles tendon ruptures or lacerations, 10 of which were neglected. They bridged the gap in the tendo-Achilles with three strips of fascia lata; a sheet of fascia lata was sutured around these grafts in a tubelike fashion, with the serosal surface outward and the seam placed anteriorly and sutured to the proximal distal stumps. A wire pull-out suture also was used. Two case reports were provided, but no other results were given, except to say that the technique gave satisfactory function and cosmetic results with no difficulty with adherent scars. Other investigators reported using fascia lata to reinforce end-to-end repairs "if deemed necessary" [56] or as one of several techniques that is used to bridge the gap in the Achilles [47,48].

Allografts.   Nellas et al [57] used two strips of freeze-dried Achilles tendon allograft to reconstruct a 4.5-cm tendon defect, following debridement of an infected primary repair. This repair was reinforced with a pull-out wire, and the patient remained in a below-knee cast for 11 weeks, followed by a period of partial weight bearing. The patient had a good functional result, although there was a reduction of peak torque compared with the uninjured side.

Synthetic materials.   The advantage of using synthetic materials is that the technique is simple and lacks donor site morbidity. Howard et al [41] used carbon fiber to repair five neglected ruptures. After a follow-up period of from 4 to 19 months, all patients had excellent results and averaged 88% plantar flexion strength compared with the opposite limb. Complications included stiffness in two patients and one delayed wound healing. Parsons et al [58] used an absorbable polymer carbon fiber composite ribbon in 48 patients who had Achilles tendon ruptures, 27 of which were chronic. The ribbon was woven through the proximal and distal stumps with six to eight passes being made to bridge the defect. A proximal tendon flap was used "at the surgeon's discretion." Postoperatively, the cast time ranged from 3 to 6 weeks; a heel lift was worn thereafter as needed. Twenty-nine patients had at least 1 year of follow-up; according to their own devised score, 86% had a good or excellent result. Complications included two reruptures, two deep infections, and three superficial infections. Amis et al [59], however, found that in sheep calcaneal tendons, carbon fiber fragmentation was associated with a poor collagen response and that with polyester implants, the neotendon was denser, more collagenous, and closely adherent. It is not known, however, whether the carbon fiber used by Howard et al and Parsons et al was similar.

Ozaki [25] reconstructed neglected ruptures in six patients—with gaps of 5 cm to 12 cm—with three layers of Marlex (USCI International, Billerica, Massachusetts) mesh (polypropylene). With a minimum of 2.4 years of follow-up, all patients showed satisfactory function and averaged 94% plantar flexion strength compared with the uninjured side; no complications were noted [60]. Levy et al [61] used a Dacron vascular graft as a tension suture material to augment a direct repair in five patients, one of whom had "a neglected rupture" even though it was only 3 weeks' postinjury. One patient was placed in a cast for 10 days postoperatively; the others began mobilization on Day 1 postoperatively with partial weight bearing at 3 weeks. Excellent results were obtained. Leiberman et al [62] reported good or excellent results in seven patients using the same material, but all of the cases were acute ruptures. Jennings and Sefton [11] used polyester tape with a Bunnel-type suture in 16 neglected ruptures. The tape was tensioned so that the ankle could just dorsiflex to neutral; this meant that the tendon gap was not always closed. A below-knee backslab was applied for 2 weeks, followed by a removable splint with weight bearing at 4 weeks. One patient required removal of the tape from around the calcaneum, one had a sural nerve injury, and three had superficial wound infections. No reruptures occurred.

Injury classification and guidelines of treatment

Kuwada [63] presented a classification scheme for Achilles tendon rupture based on 28 repairs and 102 gastrocnemius recessions. Type I injuries are partial tears that are treated with cast immobilization. Type II injury is a complete rupture with a defect that is no greater than 3 cm that is treated with end-to-end anastomosis. Type III injuries have 3-cm to 6-cm defects after debridement, and require a tendon graft flap that possibly is augmented with a synthetic graft. A defect that is greater than 6 cm is a type IV injury and requires gastrocnemius resection, a free tendon graft, or a synthetic graft.

Myerson [7] also based his treatment guidelines on the size of the tendon defect. Defects of 1 cm to 2 cm are treated with end-to-end anastomosis and posterior compartment fasciotomy. For defects of 2 cm to 5 cm, he uses a V-Y lengthening, occasionally augmented with an FHL transfer. For defects that are greater than 5 cm, he relies on an FHL tendon transfer alone or in combination with a V-Y advancement. A turndown flap can be used, but he prefers to avoid it because of the bulk of the tendon at the point at which it is passed inferiorly. We have not, however, found this to be a great problem.

Summary

Neglected Achilles tendon ruptures, although not common, are debilitating injuries. The optimal management is surgical. Many different techniques can be used to repair or reconstruct the rupture, including tendo-Achilles advancement or flap reconstruction; local tendon transfer; and autologous, autograft, or synthetic implantation. Comparison of different techniques is difficult for several reasons: (1) because of the relative rarity of the condition, the studies that are involved are retrospective and generally have small numbers; (2) patient factors can vary (eg, time from injury to repair, size of tendon defect); (3) postoperative regimes vary, from immediate mobilization to up to 3 months in plaster; and (4) reported functional outcomes also are variable, ranging from a single statement (eg, "uniformly good") to itemized functional outcome measures (none of which is validated) and dynamometer testing.

The choice of treatment is guided partly by the size of the tendon defect; however, to some extent, one can agree with Christensen [40] who, in 1953, wrote of the different operative options, "apparently all of them given good results so that, to some extent, it becomes a matter of personal preference which method one should choose."

References

[1] Lea RB, Smith L. Non-surgical treatment of tendoachillis rupture. J Bone Joint Surg 1972; 54-A(7):1392–407.
[2] Inglis AE, Sculco TP. Surgical repairs of ruptures of the tendoachillis. Clin Orthop 1981; 156:160–9.
[3] Nistor L. Surgical and non-surgical treatment of Achilles tendon rupture. A prospective randomised study. J Bone Joint Surg 1981;63-A(3):394–9.
[4] Hattrup SJ, Johnson KA. A review of ruptures of the Achilles tendon. Foot Ankle 1985;6(1): 34–8.
[5] Carden DG, Noble J, Chalmers J, et al. Rupture of the calcaneal tendon. The early and late management. J Bone Joint Surg 1987;69-B(3):416–20.
[6] Maffulli N. Current concepts review. Rupture of the Achilles tendon. J Bone Joint Surg 1999; 81-A(7):1019–36.
[7] Myerson MS. Achilles tendon ruptures. Instruct Course Lect 1999;48:219–30.
[8] Gillespie HS, George EA. Results of surgical repair of spontaneous rupture of the Achilles tendon. J Trauma 1969;9(3):247–9.
[9] Inglis AE, Scott WN, Sculco TP, et al. Ruptures of the tendoachillis. An objective assessment of surgical and non surgical treatment. J Bone Joint Surg 1976;58-A(7):990–3.
[10] Gabel S, Manol A. Neglected rupture of the Achilles tendon. Foot Ankle Int 1994;15(9):512–7.
[11] Jennings AG, Sefton GK. Chronic ruptures of the tendoachillis. Long-term results of operative management using polyester tape. J Bone Joint Surg 2002;84-B(3):361–3.

[12] Barnes MJ, Hardy AE. Delayed reconstruction of the calcaneal tendon. J Bone Joint Surg 1986;68-B:121–4.

[13] Boyden EM, Kitaoka HB, Cahalan TD, et al. Late versus early repair of Achilles tendon rupture. Clinical and biomechanical evaluation. Clin Orthop 1995;317:150–8.

[14] Mann RA, Holmes Jr GB, Seale KS, et al. Chronic ruptures of the Achilles tendon: a new technique of repair. J Bone Joint Surg 1991;73-A(2):214–9.

[15] Wilcox DK, Bohay DR, Anderson JG. Treatment of chronic Achilles tendon disorders with flexor hallucis longus tendon transfer/augmentation. Foot Ankle Int 2000;21(12):1004–10.

[16] Dalal RB, Zenios M. The flexor hallucis longus tendon transfer for chronic tendo-Achilles ruptures revisited. Ann R Coll Surg Engl 2003;85:283.

[17] Turco VJ, Spinella AJ. Achilles tendon ruptures—peroneus brevis transfer. Foot Ankle 1987;7(4):253–9.

[18] Wapner KL, Pavlock GS, Hecht PJ, et al. Repair of chronic Achilles tendon rupture with flexor hallucis longus tendon transfer. Foot Ankle 1993;14(8):443–9.

[19] Tobin WJ. Repair of neglected ruptures and severed Achilles tendon. Am Surg 1943;19:514–22.

[20] Bugg EI, Boyd BN. Repair of neglected rupture or laceration of Achilles tendon. Clin Orthop 1968;56:73–5.

[21] Rush JH. Operative repair of neglected rupture of the tendoachillis. Aust N Z J Surg 1980;50(4):420–2.

[22] Parker RG, Repinecz E. Neglected rupture of the Achilles tendon. Treatment by modified Strayer gastrocnemius resection. Journal of the American Podiatry Association 1970;69(9): 548–55.

[23] Abraham E, Pankovich AM. Neglected rupture of the Achilles tendon. Treatment by V-Y tendinous flap. J Bone Joint Surg 1975;57-A(2):253–5.

[24] Us AK, Bilgin SS, Aydin T, et al. Repair of neglected Achilles tendon ruptures: procedures and functional results. Arch Orthop Trauma Surg 1987;116:108–11.

[25] Ozaki J. Reconstruction of neglected Achilles tendon rupture with Marlex mesh. Clin Orthop 1989;238:204–8.

[26] Zadek I. Repair of old rupture of the tendo-Achilles by means of fascia. Report of a case. J Bone Joint Surg 1940;22(4):1070–1.

[27] Leitner A, Voigt C, Rahmanzadeh R. Treatment of extensive aseptic defects and old Achilles tendon ruptures: methods and case reports. Foot Ankle 1992;13(4):176–80.

[28] Platt H. Observation of some tendon repairs. BMJ 1931;1:611–5.

[29] Arner O, Lindholm A. Subcutaneous rupture of the Achilles tendon. A study of ninety two cases. Acta Chir Scand 1959;239:1–51.

[30] Conway AE. Regeneration of resected calcaneal tendon of the rabbit. Anat Rec 1967;158: 43–50.

[31] Bosworth DM. Repair of defects of the tendoachillis. J Bone Joint Surg 1956;38-A(1):111–4.

[32] Elftman H. Biomechanics of muscle with particular application to the studies of gait. J Bone Joint Surg 1966;48-A(2):363–77.

[33] Boyd EM. Intermittent claudication. A clinical study. J Bone Joint Surg 1949;31-B(3):325–55.

[34] Sutherland DH, Cooper L, Daniel D. The role of the ankle plantar flexors in normal walking. J Bone Joint Surg 1980;62-A(3):354–63.

[35] Simon SR, Mann RA, Hagy JL, et al. Role of posterior calf muscles in normal gait. J Bone Joint Surg 1978;60-A(4):465–72.

[36] Murray MP, Guten GN, Sepic SB, et al. Function of the triceps surae during gait. Compensatory mechanisms for unilateral loss. J Bone Joint Surg 1978;60-A(4):473–6.

[37] Thompson TC. A test for rupture of the tendoachillis. Acta Orthop Scand 1962;32:461–5.

[38] Harcke HT, Grissom LE, Finkelstein MS. Evaluation of the musculoskeletal system with sonography. Am J Roentgenol 1988;150:1253–61.

[39] Deutsch AL, Mink JH. Magnetic resonance imaging of musculoskeletal injuries. Radiol Clin N Am 1988;27:983–1002.

[40] Christensen I. Rupture of the Achilles tendon: analysis of 57 cases. Acta Chir Scand 1953; 106:50–60.

[41] Howard CB, Winston I, Bell W, et al. Late repair of the calcaneal tendon with carbon fibre. J Bone Joint Surg 1984;66-B(2):206–8.

[42] Kissel CG, Blacklidge OK, Crowley DL. Repair of neglected Achilles tendon ruptures—procedures and functional results. J Foot Ankle Surg 1984;33(1):46–52.

[43] Gerdes MH, Brown TD, Bell AL, et al. A flap augmentation technique for Achilles tendon repair. Post-operative strength and functional outcome. Clin Orthop 1992;28:241–6.

[44] Gilcreest E. Ruptures and tears of muscles and tendons of the lower extremity: Report of 15 cases. JAMA 1953;100:153–60.

[45] Lynn TA. Repair of the torn Achilles tendon, using the plantaris tendon as a reinforcing membrane. J Bone Joint Surg 1966;48-A(2):268–72.

[46] Schedl R, Fasol P. Achilles tendon repair with plantaris tendon compared with repair using polyglycol threads. J Trauma 1979;19(3):189–94.

[47] Hooker CH. Rupture of the tendo calcaneus. J Bone Joint Surg 1963;45-B(2):360–3.

[48] Ralston EI, Schmidt ER. Repair of the ruptured Achilles tendon. J Trauma 1971;11(1):15–21.

[49] White RK, Kraynick BM. Surgical uses of the peroneus brevis tendon. Surg Gynecol Obstet 1959;108:117–21.

[50] Teuffer AP. Traumatic ruptures of the Achilles tendon. Reconstruction by transplant and graft using the lateral peroneus brevis. Orthop Clin N Am 1974;5(1):89–93.

[51] Hansen Jr ST. Trauma to the heel cord. In: Jahss MH, editor. Disorders of the foot and ankle, vol. 3. Philadelphia: W.B. Saunders; 1991. p. 2355–60.

[52] Wapner KL, Hecht PJ, Mills Jr RH. Reconstruction of neglected Achilles tendon injury. Orthop Clin N Am 1995;26(2):249–63.

[53] St. Pierre RK, Andrews L, Allman Jr F, et al. The Cybex 2 evaluation of lateral ankle ligamentous reconstructions. Am J Sports Med 1984;12(1):52–6.

[54] Silver RL, de la Garza J, Rang M. The myth of muscle balance. A study of relative strengths and excursions of normal muscles about the foot and ankle. J Bone Joint Surg 1985;67-B(3): 432–7.

[55] Frenette JP, Jackson DW. Lacerations of the flexor hallucis longus in the young athlete. J Bone J Surg 1977;59-A(5):673–6.

[56] Distefano VJ, Nixon JE. Achilles tendon rupture: pathogenesis, diagnosis and treatment by a modified pullout wire technique. J Trauma 1972;12(8):671–7.

[57] Nellas ZJ, Loder BG, Wertheimer SJ. Reconstruction of an Achilles tendon defect utilising an Achilles tendon allograft. J Foot Ankle Surg 1996;35(2):144–8.

[58] Parsons JR, Weiss AB, Schenk RS, et al. Long-term follow-up of Achilles tendon repair with an absorbable polymer carbon fibre composite. Foot Ankle 1989;9(4):179–84.

[59] Amis AA, Campbell JR, Kempson SA, et al. Comparison of the structure of neotendons induced by implantation of carbon or polyester fibres. J Bone Joint Surg 1984;66-B(1):131–9.

[60] Kato YP, Dunn MG, Zawadsky JP, et al. Regeneration of Achilles tendon with a collagen tendon prosthesis. Results of a one-year implantation study. J Bone Joint Surg 1991;73-A(4):561–74.

[61] Levy M, Velkes S, Goldstein J, et al. A method of repair for Achilles tendon ruptures without cast immobilisation. Preliminary report. Clin Orthop 1984;187:199–204.

[62] Lieberman JR, Lozman J, Czajka J, et al. Repair of Achilles tendon ruptures with dacron vascular graft. Clin Orthop 1988;234:204–8.

[63] Kuwada GT. Classification of tendo-Achilles rupture with consideration of surgical repair techniques. J Foot Surg 1990;29(4):361–5.

ELSEVIER
SAUNDERS

Foot Ankle Clin N Am
10 (2005) 371–382

FOOT AND
ANKLE CLINICS

Achilles Tendon Rupture and Tendinopathy: Management of Complications

Jonathan S. Young, MRCS[a], Shekhar M. Kumta, MD, PhD[b],
Nicola Maffulli, MD, MS, PhD, FRCS(Orth)[a,*]

[a]*Department of Trauma and Orthopaedic Surgery, Keele University School of Medicine,
North Staffordshire Hospital, Thornburrow Drive, Hartshill, Stoke-on-Trent,
Staffordshire, ST4 7QB, UK*
[b]*Department of Orthopaedics and Traumatology, The Chinese University of Hong Kong,
Prince of Wales Hospital, 30–32 Ngan Shing Street, Shatin, New Territories, Hong Kong*

Ailments of the Achilles tendon are on the increase and present in athletic and sedentary patients [1]. The management of tendinopathy and rupture is not codified; Achilles tendon rupture and tendinopathy can be managed conservatively or surgically. Tackling the complications that arise from the management of these conditions provides a formidable challenge to the surgeon. Rupture, rerupture, disordered scarring with potential keloid formation, nerve damage (especially the sural nerve), poor healing, infection, bleeding and hematoma formation, wound dehiscence, deep vein thrombosis (DVT), and loss of function have been reported [1–4]. This article gives an up-to-date account on our personal views of managing complications following Achilles tendon rupture, tendinopathy, and delayed rupture.

Complications following rupture of the Achilles tendon

The Achilles tendon is the most commonly ruptured tendon in the human body [5] and its incidence is increasing [6]. Surgery for Achilles tendon rup-

---

* Corresponding author.
E-mail address: n.maffulli@keele.ac.uk (N. Maffulli).

1083-7515/05/$ – see front matter © 2005 Elsevier Inc. All rights reserved.
doi:10.1016/j.fcl.2005.01.004
foot.theclinics.com

tures can be performed using open or percutaneous techniques, whereas neglected ruptures are managed most often by open procedures, with reinforcement of the tendon or grafting [7]. The increasing incidence of ruptures of the Achilles tendon may be a result of increasing popularity in sport [8]. Ruptures are more common in men and on the left side [6,9]. Their etiology is unclear. Histologic evidence of collagen degeneration in ruptured tendons is present before rupture [10]. Sport, in addition to normal daily activities, might lead to microtears and intratendinous degenerative changes [11]. The Achilles tendon has a poor blood supply throughout its length, as shown by the small number of blood vessels per cross-sectional area. Poor vascularity may prevent adequate tissue repair following trauma and lead to further weakening of the tendon [12].

The diagnosis of ruptured Achilles tendon usually is not difficult for experienced surgeons [7,13]. Patients typically report a snapping sensation at the posterior aspect of the ankle in association with pain and inability to weight bear. On examination, a palpable gap can be appreciated. In Simmond's test, the patient lies prone on the couch with the feet over the edge. When squeezing the calf, an intact Achilles tendon produces plantarflexion of the ankle against gravity [14]. In Matles' test, with the patient lying prone in the bed, both legs are flexed to 90° until the tibiae are perpendicular to the floor. The nonruptured side will remain in some degree of plantar flexion, whereas the ruptured side will lie in neutral or dorsiflex [15]. If there is uncertainty from clinical tests (perhaps in the case of neglected rupture, where fibrous tissue may fill the gap), ultrasound (US) or MRI scanning should be considered [16,17].

Complications of Achilles tendon ruptures can be divided into complications of conservative management, complications of surgical management, and complications of conservative and surgical management. There is ongoing debate on how to deal with an early acute rupture of the Achilles tendon. The management options are surgical or nonsurgical; surgical management involves open or percutaneous methods. Management, to some degree, depends on the time of presentation, the patient's degree of athleticism, age, fitness, and personal preference. The preference of the surgeon also plays a factor. There is no established protocol for the management of ruptures [1,18]. Management of Achilles tendon ruptures should allow the tendon to heal and return the patient to an acceptable functional level. Factors, such as age, occupation, and recreational activities, should be taken into account when counseling patients. Nestorson et al [19] examined the functional ability after Achilles tendon rupture in 25 patients who were older than 65 years. Fourteen were managed surgically and 10 were managed conservatively; one patient received no treatment. Only 9 patients returned to their previous activity level, and 11 patients had at least one complication. Achilles tendon rupture in this age group reduces lower limb function; complications were common following surgical and nonsurgical management. Surgical repair may not be beneficial, on average, in patients who are older than 65 years.

Complications following conservative management of ruptured Achilles tendon

Wallace et al [20] reported excellent results with conservative management using a hard cast for 1 month before switching to a functional brace for another month. In contrast, Persson and Wredmark [21] showed that 7 of 27 patients had a rerupture, and an additional 7 patients were not satisfied with the result of conservative management. Conservative management may lengthen the tendon and alter its function [22]. This may need surgical correction [23], and can be avoided in the first place if surgery is performed [1]. Haggmark et al [24] highlighted the functional problems that are associated with Achilles tendon rupture. They followed 23 patients for 3 to 5 years; 15 had an open repair and 8 were managed nonoperatively. The latter group had significantly impaired dynamic calf muscle function compared with patients who were managed operatively, in whom no such impairment was shown. Many investigators believe that aside from the functional problems of conservative management, there also is a greater rerupture rate. Wong et al [25] reported a rerupture rate of 10.7% for conservative management of rupture. Lo et al [26] had an overall rerupture rate of 2.8% for patients who were managed operatively and 11. 7% for patients who were managed nonoperatively ($P < .001$).

Complications following surgical management of ruptured Achilles tendon

Surgical management significantly reduces the risk of Achilles tendon rerupture, but increases the risk of infection when compared with conservative management [27]. Arner and Lindholm [28] reported a 24% complication rate in 86 operative repairs, including one death from pulmonary embolism. Open repair caused 20 times more minor to moderate complications than conservative management; however, there was no significant difference in the frequency of major complications [26]. Open repair can be performed in various ways using simple end-to-end repairs (Bunnell/Kessler), or more complex techniques with fascial reinforcement or tendon grafts [29,30]. There is no significant evidence to support more complex primary repairs in acute Achilles tendon ruptures [31]. The results of open repair vary markedly [28,32]. These differences are likely to be multi-factorial and may result from subtle variations in technique, degree of experience of the operating surgeon, the type of suture material used, and the location of incision.

Percutaneous repair [33] is a compromise between open surgery and conservative management, although the early reports outlined an increased risk of rerupture and of damage to the sural nerve. Ma and Griffith [33] reported an excellent success rate with no reruptures and two minor complications. Some studies demonstrated that the rate of rerupture after percutaneous repair is greater than that after open operative procedures [34,35]. More recent studies that compared the two repair techniques showed similar results, with no difference in rerupture rate between percutaneous and open repair [36]. That study, however, showed a significantly greater rate of infective wound complications using open repair [36].

Compartment syndrome is rare following ruptured Achilles tendon [37]. Many surgeons use a tourniquet in the repair of Achilles tendon. Although usually safe, there have been cases of compartment syndrome following tourniquet use for lower limb surgery [38]. Any pre- and postoperative swelling or stiffness of the muscles in the operation area should be noted, even if the recommended time or pressure limits are not exceeded [38]. If the diagnosis of compartment syndrome is made, fasciotomy should be performed promptly.

Muscle wasting is a complication of subcutaneous rupture of the Achilles tendon. CT and morphologic studies showed a significant decrease in calf muscle cross-sectional area and hypotrophy of the soleus muscle in seven athletes who had surgery for Achilles tendon rupture [39]. Prompt surgical management of ruptures, with cast changes several times during the period of immobilization and with tension maintained on the muscle, is an effective regimen for this injury. Wong et al [25] documented quicker functional recovery with open repair, and also noted a trend to improved functional outcome with early mobilization. Early weight bearing and early mobilization are not detrimental to the outcome of repair after acute rupture of the Achilles tendon, and shorten the time needed for rehabilitation [40].

If a longitudinal incision is used in open repair of the Achilles tendon, it passes through poorly-vascularized skin [41], with the potential for poorly healing wounds. Even defects that are less than 1 cm^2 take a long time to heal. Wounds that break down need coverage, because tendons that are left exposed undergo desiccation and secondary adhesions [42]. Local or free flap coverage may achieve this if the lesion is not responsive to conservative management. Local flap coverage can be in the form of medial plantar flap, posterior tibial reverse flow flap, or peroneal reverse flow island flap, depending on the site of defect [43]. This is advantageous in restricting the morbidity of the leg that originally was operated on; if a local flap fails, a free flap still can be considered. We reported a high success rate with local flaps in defects that were less than 2.5 × 2.5 cm [43]; however, complications have to be recognized early and should receive expedient appropriate management.

A free flap is appropriate in larger defects. A radial artery free flap [44], tensor fascia latae perforator flap [45], latissimus dorsi free flap [46], lateral arm free flap [47], peroneal artery free flap [48], temporal artery fascial free flap [49], and free quadriceps bone tendon graft [50] have been used in this situation. The choice of flap depends largely on the surgeon and the patient's wishes. It should be explained to the patients that they will have a residual scar at the site from which the flap was harvested, with potential functional and cosmetic problems (Table 1).

Less common complications of Achilles tendon rupture include peritendinous calcifications after open repair [53]. These can be managed conservatively or operatively. Kraus et al [53] elected for operative management with postoperative

Table 1
Type of flap used to manage skin loss following surgery to the Achilles tendon (in chronologic order)

Authors	Number of operations	Type of flap
Kumta and Maffuli, 2003 [43]	4	Reverse pedicle posterior tibial fasciocutaneous flap
Upton et al, 1994 [49]	15	Free fascial flap; 13 parietotemporal, 2 forearm
Leppilahti et al, 1996 [53]	4	3 radial artery, 1 lateral arm flap
Berthe et al, 1998 [47]	1	Lateral arm flap
Ademoglu et al, 2001 [3]	4	3 lateral arm, 1 radial artery
Mugdal et al, 2000 [55]	1 (2-stage)	Free quadriceps bone tendon graft with fascial gastrocnemius flap
Chun et al, 2001 [44]	2	Radial artery
Delier et al, 2001 [45]	5	Tensor fascia latae
Kumta and Maffuli, 2003 [43]	11	6 medial plantar, 4 peroneal reverse flow, 1 posterior tibial reverse flow
Kumta and Maffuli, 2003 [43]	10	3 gastrocnemius flap, 4 lateral foot flap, 2 superior medial malleolus, 1 sural neural flap

chemical prophylaxis. At 1 year follow-up, the patient was pain-free. In general, we adopt a conservative regimen in these patients, with an expectant attitude. Ossification of the Achilles tendon is rare, and is distinct from the more frequent intratendinous calcification. Achilles tendon ossification is more common in men and usually is associated with previous surgery or trauma to the tendon [51,52, 54,56]. Heavy work, bilateral occurrence, repetitive microtrauma to the Achilles tendon and some predisposition are causative factors [67]. An ossified Achilles tendon can fracture, which functionally results in a rupture [68].

Another complication of Achilles tendon rupture is a cavus foot following failed repair [57]. This probably arises from the decrease in push-off being compensated by the intrinsic and extrinsic muscles of the foot. Patients have increased passive dorsiflexion on the affected side with clawing of the toes, limping, pain, and function loss.

Complications of conservative and surgical management of ruptured Achilles tendon

DVT may follow surgical and conservative management [58], and has several documented risk factors (eg, age, immobility, malignancy, blood dyscrasias, pregnancy, previous DVT, and prolonged surgery). It is not common following Achilles tendon repair. Arner and Lindholm [28] reported two DVTs in 86 patients following open repair of Achilles tendon. One of these patients developed a pulmonary embolism (PE), and subsequently died. DVT and associated PE can be minimized by early mobilization, making sure that the patient receives appropriate DVT prophylaxis [59]. DVT in the affected leg is difficult to diagnose, because patients often are in an equinus plaster for some weeks. Careful history taking and re-examination of the affected leg in and out of plaster on a regular basis are recommended. Achilles tendon operations can be performed under regional nerve blocks, which would avoid potentially prolonged immobilization and the risks of general anesthesia, including DVT. If there is a suspicion of DVT, D dimers and an urgent US scan of the affected leg should be requested. If positive, the patient should be anticoagulated [60]. In PE, the patient also needs a ventilation perfusion scan, spiral CT, or pulmonary angiography [61], as well as anticoagulation [60].

Rerupture is a complication of surgical and conservative management, but it generally is more common with conservative management [26]. Early careful ankle mobilization and full weight bearing after primary Achilles tendon repair does not increase the risk of rerupture [62].

Delayed presentation of rupture of the Achilles tendon

Delayed presentation of a ruptured Achilles tendon is a more challenging problem for the surgeon and the patient. The tendon ends often are retracted, and they will need to be freshened, which leaves a larger gap [7]. This poses problems for the patient regarding function and morbidity—because the patient already has a functional deficit from the delayed diagnosis—and a more extensive open operation must be performed. The aim in delayed rupture is to achieve good skin healing with a functional muscle tendon unit. Different open techniques have been used to bridge the gap effectively, including V-Y gastrocnemius flap [63] and flexor hallucis longus tendon transfer [64]. Transfer of the flexor hallucis longus tendon showed good results, but there is the potential for loss of push from the hallux while sprinting which affects function in athletes [64].

Perez-Teuffer [65] used the peroneus brevis tendon in delayed Achilles tendon ruptures. Aside from functional problems, complications include wound hematoma and sural nerve injury. These risks can be minimized with careful hemostasis, and appropriate soft tissue handling. For example, maintaining thick skin flaps throughout the procedure helps to avoid wound breakdown. Although the original description of the technique involved a lateral approach, we advocate performing this procedure through a medial incision, which prevents sural nerve injury [7]. Pintore et al [66] highlighted the morbidity that is associated with delayed ruptures. In a single-center, single-surgeon study of 49 patients who had a fresh (4 women and 23 men) or neglected (1 woman and 21 men) Achilles tendon rupture, patients generally were satisfied with the procedure. Those who had a neglected rupture tended to have a greater rate of postoperative complications, greater loss of isokinetic strength at high speeds, and greater loss of calf circumference. The management of acute and neglected subcutaneous tears of the Achilles tendon by peroneus tendon transfer is safe but technically demanding. It affords good recovery, even in patients who have a neglected rupture of 6 weeks' to 9 months' duration. Patients who have a neglected rupture are at a slightly greater risk of postoperative complications and their ankle plantar flexion strength can be reduced.

Complications following Achilles tendinopathy

Excessive repetitive overload of the Achilles tendon is the main pathologic stimulus that leads to tendinopathy [67,68]. This condition, as in the case of a ruptured Achilles tendon, can be managed conservatively or surgically. Conservative management involves intensive physiotherapy with eccentric exercises [69]. Kvist and Kvist [70] argued that conservative management is unsatisfactory. Tatari at al [71] investigated the effect of heparin on Achilles tendon injury and concluded that it had a degenerative effect on the tendon and should not be used in the treatment of Achilles tendinopathy.

Anti-inflammatories are beneficial in the initial inflammatory response and its symptoms, but may have detrimental effects during the healing phase [67,72]. Riley et al [73] investigated the effects of some commonly used nonsteroidal anti-inflammatory drugs (NSAIDs) on human tendon. Diclofenac and aceclofenac had no significant effect on tendon cell proliferation or glycosaminoglycan synthesis. Indomethacin and naproxen inhibited cell proliferation in patella tendons and inhibited glycosaminoglycan synthesis in digital flexor and patella tendons. If applicable to the in vivo situation, these NSAIDs should be used with caution in the treatment of pain after tendon injury and surgery. Almekinders et al [74] suggest that NSAIDs may have negative effects during the proliferative phase of healing, because they were associated with decreased DNA synthesis; however, NSAIDs may be beneficial in the maturation and remodeling phase because they stimulated protein synthesis. Long-term use of these drugs has implications in peptic ulcer formation and can lead to transient renal impairment [75]. A careful history regarding dyspepsia should be taken before prescribing; if long-term use is required, monitoring of electrolytes is recommended [75,76].

The use of steroids for tendinopathy is controversial. Koenig et al [77] investigated the effects of intratendinous glucocorticoid injection for acute Achilles tendinopathy in five patients. They hypothesized that the intratendinous hyperemia that was seen with US color Doppler represented an inflammatory response. Six tendons in five patients were evaluated with gray-scale US and color Doppler before and after US-guided intratendinous glucocorticoid injection. Pain and color Doppler activity decreased during a mean follow-up of 182 days. Intratendinous glucocorticoid injections seem to have a marked effect on symptoms and color Doppler findings, which may be taken as an indication of an inflammatory component in the disease. It should be kept in mind that the patients who were reported in this study presented acutely, and are not representative of the patients who have chronic Achilles tendinopathy that are seen commonly in tertiary referral practices.

Corticosteroids have been administered for tendinopathy, but evidence of their effectiveness is lacking and there is no good scientific reason to support their use. Intratendinous injections of corticosteroids in patients who have established Achilles tendinopathy are to be avoided [67]. Oral and peritendinous steroid injections have been associated with Achilles tendon rupture [78,79]. Newnham et al [78] reported a series of 10 patients who attended a respiratory outpatient clinic, were taking oral corticosteroids, and subsequently ruptured their Achilles tendon in the course of 12 years. Achilles tendon rupture is a complication of corticosteroid treatment. Speed [80] reviewed the literature on corticosteroid injections involving tendinopathies and concluded that there was no good evidence to support corticosteroid injections. Gill et al [81], in a retrospective cohort study of 83 patients, established the safety of low-volume injections of corticosteroids for the management of Achilles tendinopathy when the needle is inserted carefully into the peritendinous space under direct fluoroscopic visualization. In this study, although 23 patients (27.7%) did not report any improvement, only 3 patients (3.6%) believed that their condition was worse.

In 432 consecutive patients who were managed surgically for chronic Achilles tendinopathy that was resistant to conservative management, Paavola et al [82] documented an 11% complication rate. These complications included 14 skin edge necroses, 11 superficial wound infections, 5 seroma formations, 5 hematomas, 5 fibrotic reactions or scar formations, 4 sural nerve irritations, 1 new partial rupture, and 1 deep vein thrombosis. Fourteen patients required another surgery. Most patients who had a complication healed and returned to their preinjury levels of activity. Surgeons should be aware of the possibility of postoperative complications and use appropriate surgical techniques.

Summary

Achilles tendon rupture and tendinopathy and the associated complications of conservative and surgical management present many challenges. Good clinical acumen, knowledge of management options, the appropriate surgery, and good soft tissue handling helps to avoid complications, but they do occur, even in experienced hands. Most complications resolve on their own using conservative management; however, for those that do not, aggressive and prompt management by experienced physicians is needed.

References

[1] Maffulli N. Rupture of the Achilles tendon. J Bone Joint Surg Am 1999;81-A:1019–36.
[2] Cinotti A, Massari L, Traina GC, et al. The echographic and clinical follow-up of pa-
    tients operated on for subcutaneous rupture of the Achilles tendon. Radiol Med (Torino) 1996;
    91:28–32.
[3] Ademoglu Y, Ozerkan F, Ada A, et al. Reconstruction of skin and tendon defects from
    wound complications after Achilles tendon rupture. J Foot Ankle Surg 2001;40(3):158–65.

[4] Dalton G, Wapner K, Hecht P. Complications of Achilles and posterior tibial tendon surgeries. Clin Orthop 2001;391:133–9.

[5] Jozsa L, Kvist M, Balint J, et al. The role of recreational sports activity in Achilles tendon rupture: a clinical, patho-anatomical and sociological study of 292 cases. Am J Sports Med 1989;17:338–43.

[6] Maffulli N, Waterston SW, Squair J, et al. Changing incidence of Achilles tendon rupture in Scotland: a 15-year study. Clin J Sport Med 1999;9:157–60.

[7] McClelland D, Maffulli N. The management of neglected ruptures of the Achilles tendon: Reconstruction with peroneus brevis tendon transfer. The Surgeon 2004;2:209–13.

[8] Leppilahti J, Puranen J, Orava S. Incidence of Achilles tendon rupture. Acta Orthop Scand 1996;67:277–9.

[9] Stein SR, Luekens CA. Abstract methods and rationale for closed treatment of Achilles tendon ruptures. Am J Sports Med 1976;4:162–9.

[10] Arner O, Lindholm A, Orell SR. Histologic changes in subcutaneous rupture of the Achilles tendon; a study of 74 cases. Acta Chir Scand 1958–59;116:484–90.

[11] Fox J, Blazina M, Jobe F, et al. Degeneration and rupture of the Achilles tendon. Clin Orthop 1975;107:221–4.

[12] Ahmed IM, Lagopoulos M, McConnell P, et al. Blood supply of the Achilles tendon. J Orthop Res 1998;16:591–6.

[13] Maffulli N. The clinical diagnosis of subcutaneous tear of the Achilles tendon. A prospective study in 174 patients. Am J Sports Med 1998;26:266–70.

[14] Simmonds FA. The diagnosis of the ruptured Achilles tendon. Practioner 1957;179:56–8.

[15] Matles AL. Rupture of the tendo Achilles. Another diagnostic sign. Bull Hosp Joint Dis 1975;36:48–51.

[16] Crass JR, Craig EV, Feinberg SB. Clinical significance of sonographic findings in the abnormal but intact rotator cuff: a preliminary report. J Clin Ultrasound 1988;16:625–34.

[17] Kabbani YM, Mayer DP. Magnetic resonance imaging of tendon pathology about the foot and ankle. Part II. Tendon ruptures. J Am Podiatr Med Assoc 1993;83:466–8.

[18] Leppilahti J, Orava S. Total Achilles tendon rupture. A review. Sports Med 1998;25:79–100.

[19] Nestorson J, Movin T, Moller M, et al. Function after Achilles tendon rupture in the elderly: 25 patients older than 65 years followed for 3 years. Acta Orthop Scand 2000;71:64–8.

[20] Wallace RG, Traynor IE, Kernohan WG, et al. Combined conservative and orthotic management of acute ruptures of the Achilles tendon. J Bone Joint Surg Am 2004;86:1198–202.

[21] Persson A, Wredmark T. The treatment of total ruptures of the Achilles tendon by plaster immobilisation. Internat Orthop 1979;3:149–52.

[22] Bohnsack M, Ruhmann O, Kirsch L, Wirth CJ. Surgical shortening of the Achilles tendon for correction of elongation following healed conservatively treated Achilles tendon rupture. Z Orthop Ihre Grenzgeb 2000;138:501–5.

[23] Soma C, Mandelbaum B. Repair of acute Achilles tendon ruptures. Orthop Clin North Am 1976;7:241–6.

[24] Haggmark T, Liedberg H, Eriksson E, et al. Calf muscle atrophy and muscle function after non-operative vs operative treatment of Achilles tendon ruptures. Orthopedics 1986;9:160–4.

[25] Wong J, Barrass V, Maffulli N. Quantitative review of operative and nonoperative management of Achilles tendon ruptures. Am J Sports Med 2002;30:565–75.

[26] Lo IK, Kirkley A, Nonweiler B, et al. Operative versus nonoperative treatment of acute Achilles tendon ruptures: a quantitative review. Clin J Sport Med 1997;7:207–11.

[27] Bhandari M, Guyatt GH, Siddiqui F, et al. Treatment of acute Achilles tendon ruptures: a systematic overview and metaanalysis. Clin Orthop 2002;400:190–200.

[28] Arner O, Lindholm A. Subcutaneous rupture of the Achilles tendon. A study of 92 cases. Acta Chir Scand 1959;116(Supp 239):1–5.

[29] Bosworth D. Repair of defects in the tendo Achilles. J Bone Joint Surg Am 1956;38:111–4.

[30] Lynn T. Repair of torn Achilles tendon, using the plantaris tendon as a reinforcing membrane. J Bone Joint Surg Am 1966;48:268–72.

[31] Jessing P, Hansen E. Surgical treatment of 102 tendo Achilles ruptures—suture or tenoplasty? Acta Chir Scand 1975;141:370–7.

[32] Soldatis J, Goodfellow D, Wilber J. End to end operative repair of Achilles tendon rupture. Am J Sports Med 1997;25:90–5.

[33] Ma GWC, Griffith TG. Percutaneous repair of acute closed ruptured Achilles tendon. A new technique. Clin Orthop 1977;128:247–55.

[34] Aracil J, Lozano J, Torro V, et al. Percutaneous suture of Achilles tendon ruptures. Foot Ankle 1992;13:350–1.

[35] Bradley J, Tibone J. Percutaneous and open surgical repairs of Achilles tendon ruptures. A comparative study. Am J Sports Med 1990;18:188–95.

[36] Lim J, Dalal R, Waseem M. Percutaneous vs. open repair of the ruptured Achilles tendon. A prospective study. Foot Ankle Int 2001;22:559–68.

[37] Reed J, Hiemstra LA. Anterior compartment syndrome following an Achilles tendon repair: an unusual complication. Clin J Sport Med 2004;14:237–41.

[38] Hirvensalo E, Tuominen H, Lapinsuo M, et al. Compartment syndrome of the lower limb caused by a tourniquet: a report of two cases. J Orthop Trauma 1992;6:469–72.

[39] Haggmark T, Eriksson E. Hypotrophy of the soleus muscle in a man after Achilles tendon rupture. Discussion of findings obtained by computed tomography and morphologic studies. Am J Sports Med 1979;7(2):121–6.

[40] Maffulli N, Tallon C, Wong J, et al. Early weightbearing and ankle mobilization after open repair of acute midsubstance tears of the Achilles tendon. Am J Sports Med 2003;31:692–700.

[41] Haertsch PA. The blood supply of the skin of the leg: a post-mortem investigation. Br J Plast Surg 1981;34:470–7.

[42] Leung PC, Hung LK, Leung KS. Use of medial plantar flap in soft tissue replacement around the heel region. Foot Ankle 1988;8:327–30.

[43] Kumta SM, Maffulli N. Local flap coverage for soft tissue defects following open repair of Achilles tendon rupture. Acta Orthop Belg 2003;69:59–66.

[44] Chun J, Margoles S, Birnbaum J. Radial forearm free flap for salvage of Achilles tendon repair wounds. J Reconstr Microsurg 2000;16:519–23.

[45] Deiler S, Pfadenhauer A, Widmann J, et al. Tensor fasciae latae perforator flap for recon-struction of composite Achilles tendon defects with skin and vascularized fasciae. Plast Reconstr Surg 2001;106(2):342–9.

[46] Ronel D, Newman M, Gayle L, et al. Recent advances in the reconstruction of complex Achilles tendon defects. Microsurgery 2004;24:18–23.

[47] Berthe J, Toussaint D, Coessens B. One stage reconstruction of an infected skin and Achilles tendon defect with a composite distally planned lateral arm flap. Plast Reconstr Surg 1998;102:1618–22.

[48] Yoshimura M, Imura S, Shimamura K, et al. Peroneal flap for reconstruction in the extremity: Preliminary report. Plastic Reconstr Ssurg 1984;74:402–9.

[49] Upton J, Baker T, Shoen S, et al. Fascial flap coverage of Achilles tendon defects. Plast Reconstr Surg 1995;95:1056–61.

[50] Mudgal C, Martin T, Wilson M. Reconstruction of Achilles tendon defect with a free quadriceps bone-tendon graft without anastomosis. Foot Ankle Int 2000;21:10–3.

[51] Upton J, Ferraro N, Healy G, et al. The use of prefabricated fascial flaps for lining of the oral and nasal cavities. Plast Reconstr Surg 1994;94(5):573–9.

[52] Leppilahti J, Kaarela O, Teerikangas H, et al. Free tissue coverage of wound complications following Achilles tendon rupture surgery. Clin Orthop 1996;328:171–6.

[53] Kraus R, Horas U, Stahl J, et al. Operative treatment of extended peritendinous calcifications after open Achilles tendon repair-a case report. Unfallchirug 2003;106:680–2.

[54] Sobel E, Giorgini R, Hilfer J, et al. Ossification of a ruptured Achilles tendon: a case report in a diabetic patient. J Foot Ankle Surg 2002;41:330–4.

[55] Hatori M, Matsuda M, Kokubun S. Ossification of Achilles tendon—report of three cases. Arch Orthop Trauma Surg 2002;122:414–7.

[56] Aksoy MC, Surat A. Fracture of the ossified Achilles tendon. Acta Orthop Belg 1998;64:418–21.

[57] Fortems Y, Victor J. Development of cave foot deformity in failed repair of Achilles tendon. Arch Orthop Trauma Surg 1993;112:121–3.

[58] Silbersack Y, Taute B, Hein W, et al. Prevention of deep-vein thrombosis after total hip and knee replacement. Low-molecular-weight heparin in combination with intermittent pneumatic compression. J Bone Joint Surg Br 2004;86:809–12.

[59] Volpicello C. Pulmonary embolism after repair of a traumatic Achilles tendon rupture. AORN J 1996;64(4):599–601.

[60] Cosmi B, Palareti G. Oral anticoagulant therapy in venous thromboembolism. Semin Vasc Med 2003;3:303–14.

[61] Buksa M, Gerc V. New aspects in the diagnosis of pulmonary embolism. Med Arh 2004;58: 47–50.

[62] Speck M, Klaue K. Early full weightbearing and functional treatment after surgical repair of acute Achilles tendon rupture. Am J Sports Med 1998;26:789–93.

[63] Abraham E, Pankovich AM. Neglected rupture of Achilles tendon. Treatment by V-Y tendinous flap. J Bone Joint Surg Am 1975;57:253–5.

[64] Wapner KL, Pavlock GS, Hecht PJ, et al. Repair of chronic Achilles tendon rupture with flexor hallucis longus tendon transfer. Foot Ankle 1993;14:443–9.

[65] Perez-Teuffer A. A traumatic rupture of the Achilles tendon. Reconstruction by transplant and graft using the lateral peroneus brevis. Orthop Clin N Am 1974;5:89–93.

[66] Pintore E, Barra V, Pintore R, et al. Peroneus brevis tendon transfer in neglected tears of the Achilles tendon. J Trauma 2001;50:71–8.

[67] Maffulli N, Kader D. Tendinopathy of tendo Achilles. J Bone Joint Surg Br 2002;84:1–8.

[68] Kvist M. Achilles tendon overuse injuries [thesis]. Ann Univ Turku 1991;87:1–121.

[69] Cook J, Khan K, Purdam C. Achilles tendinopathy. Man Ther 2002;7:121–30.

[70] Kvist H, Kvist M. The operative treatment of chronic calcaneal paratendinous. J Bone Joint Surg Br 1980;62:353–7.

[71] Tatari H, Kosay C, Baran O, et al. Effect of heparin on tendon degeneration: an experimental study on rats. Knee Surg Sports Traumatol Arthrosc 2001;9:247–53.

[72] Almekinders LC. Anti-inflammatory treatment of muscular injuries in sport. An update of recent studies. Sports Med 1999;28:383–8.

[73] Riley GP, Cox M, Harrall RL, et al. Inhibition of tendon cell proliferation and matrix glycosaminoglycan synthesis by non-steroidal anti-inflammatory drugs in vitro. J Hand Surg [Br] 2001;26:224–8.

[74] Almekinders LC, Baynes AJ, Bracey LW. An in vitro investigation into the effects of repetitive motion and nonsteroidal antiinflammatory medication on human tendon fibroblasts. Am J Sports Med 1995;23:119–23.

[75] Lee A, Cooper MC, Craig JC, et al. Effects of nonsteroidal anti-inflammatory drugs on postoperative renal function in adults with normal renal function. Cochrane Database Syst Rev 2004;(2):CD002765.

[76] Arroyo MT, Forne M, de Argila CM, et al. The prevalence of peptic ulcer not related to Helicobacter pylori or non-steroidal anti-inflammatory drug use is negligible in southern Europe. Helicobacter 2004;9:249–54.

[77] Koenig MJ, Torp-pedersen S, Qvistgaard E, et al. Preliminary results of colour Doppler-guided intratendinous glucocorticoid injection for Achilles tendonitis in five patients. Scand J Med Sci Sports 2004;14:100–6.

[78] Newnham D, Douglas J, Legge J, et al. Achilles tendon rupture: an underrated complication of corticosteroid treatment. Thorax 1991;46:853–4.

[79] Unverferth L, Olix M. The effect of local steroid injections on tendon. J Sports Med 1973;1: 31–7.

[80] Speed CA. Corticosteroid injections in tendon lesions. BMJ 2001;323:382–6.

[81] Gill SS, Gelbke MK, Mattson SL, et al. Fluoroscopically guided low-volume peritendinous corticosteroid injection for Achilles tendinopathy. A safety study. J Bone Joint Surg Am 2004;86-A:802–6.

[82] Paavola M, Orava S, Leppilahti J, et al. Chronic Achilles tendon overuse injury: complications after surgical treatment. An analysis of 432 consecutive patients. Am J Sport Med 2000; 28:77–82.

ELSEVIER
SAUNDERS

Foot Ankle Clin N Am
10 (2005) 383–397

FOOT AND
ANKLE CLINICS

The Future: Rehabilitation, Gene Therapy, Optimization of Healing

Pankaj Sharma, MBBS, MRCS[a,b],
Nicola Maffulli, MD, MS, PhD, FRCS(Orth)[b,*]

[a]Department of Trauma and Orthopaedic Surgery, Highcroft, Romsey Road, Wessex Deanery,
Winchester, SO22 5DH, UK
[b]Department of Trauma and Orthopaedics, Keele University School of Medicine, Thornburrow Drive,
Hartshill, Stoke-on-Trent ST4 7QB, UK

Tendons transmit force generated by muscle to bone, and exhibit high mechanical strength, good flexibility, and an optimal level of elasticity to perform their unique role [1–3]. Tendons are viscoelastic tissues that display stress relaxation and creep [4,5].

The mechanical behavior of collagen is dependent on the number and types of intra- and intermolecular bonds [4,5]. At rest, collagen fibers and fibrils display a crimped configuration [6]. At less than a 4% strain, human tendons behave in an elastic fashion—as a result of intramolecular sliding of collagen triple helices—and return to their original length when unloaded [7–9]. Microscopic failure occurs when the strain exceeds 4%; beyond 8% to 10% strain, macroscopic failure occurs as a result of intrafibril damage by molecular slippage [2,10,11]. Complete failure then occurs rapidly, and the fibers recoil into a tangled bud at the ruptured end.

The tensile strength of tendons is related to their thickness and to their collagen content; a tendon with an cross-sectional area of 1 cm^2 can support 500 kg to 1000 kg [12,13]. In the human Achilles tendon, forces of 9 kN, corresponding to 12.5 times body weight, have been recorded during running [14–16].

Following injury, remodeling occurs after a period of up to 2 years. Despite active remodeling, the biochemical and mechanical properties of healed tendon tissue never match those of intact tendons. The final tensile strength of a healed

* Corresponding author.
E-mail address: n.maffulli@keele.ac.uk (N. Maffulli).

tendon may be reduced by as much as 30% [17]. A possible reason for this may be the absence of mechanical loading during the period of immobilization. This article considers the stages of tendon healing, and reviews possible strategies for optimizing tendon healing and repair.

Tendon healing

Tendon healing studies have been performed predominantly on transected animal tendons or ruptured human tendons; their relevance to tendinopathic and ruptured human tendons remains unclear. Tendon healing occurs in three overlapping phases. In the initial inflammatory phase, erythrocytes and inflammatory cells, particularly neutrophils, enter the site of injury. In the first 24 hours, monocytes and macrophages predominate, and phagocytosis of necrotic materials occurs. Vasoactive and chemotactic factors are released which leads to increased vascular permeability, initiation of angiogenesis, stimulation of tenocyte proliferation, and recruitment of more inflammatory cells [18,19]. Tenocytes gradually migrate to the wound and type III collagen synthesis is initiated [20].

After a few days, the regenerative stage begins. Synthesis of type III collagen peaks during this stage, which lasts for a few weeks. Water content and glycosaminoglycan concentrations remain high during this stage [20].

Remodeling commences approximately 6 weeks after the injury, with decreased cellularity and decreased collagen and glycosaminoglycan synthesis. This phase can be divided into a consolidation stage and a maturation stage [21]. The former commences at about 6 weeks and continues for up to 4 weeks. In this period, the repair tissue changes from cellular to fibrous. Tenocyte metabolism remains high during this period, and tenocytes and collagen fibers become aligned in the direction of stress [22,23]. A greater proportion of type I collagen is synthesized during this stage [24]. After 10 weeks from the injury, maturation starts to take place, with gradual change of fibrous tissue to scarlike tendon tissue [22,25]. Increased covalent bonding between collagen fibers results in greater tensile strength and stiffness of the repair tissue [26]. The maturation stage continues for up to a year; however, during the latter half of this stage, tenocyte metabolism and tendon vascularity decline [27].

Epitenon tenoblasts initiate the repair process through proliferation and migration [28–30]. Healing in severed tendons can be affected by tenocytes from the epitenon alone, without relying on adhesions for vascularity or cellular support [31,32]. Internal tenocytes contribute to the intrinsic repair process and secrete larger and more mature collagen than do epitenon cells [33]. Despite this, epitenon and tendon tenocytes synthesize collagen during repair, and different cells probably produce collagen at different time points. Initially, collagen is produced by epitenon cells, whereas endotenon cells synthesize collagen later [34–38]. The relative contribution of each cell type may be influenced by the type of trauma sustained, anatomic position, presence of a synovial sheath, and the amount of postrepair motion stress [39].

Intrinsic healing generally results in improved biomechanics and fewer complications [40]. In extrinsic healing, scar tissue results in adhesion formation which disrupts tendon gliding [41]. Different healing patterns may predominate in particular locations; extrinsic healing prevails in torn rotator cuffs [42].

Cytokines are small proteins that evoke cellular responses by engaging specific cell-surface receptors [43]. A complex system exists, whereby cytokines may have multiple dose-dependent effects, and act synergistically with other cytokines. The importance of growth factors as regulators of the phases of tendon healing has been well-established [43–48]. Wounding and inflammation provoke the release of growth factors from platelets, polymorphonuclear leukocytes, and macrophages [44,45,48]. These growth factors induce neovascularization and chemotaxis, and stimulate tenocyte proliferation and collagen synthesis [49,50].

Optimization strategies

Current management strategies, such as nonsteroidal anti-inflammatory drugs or corticosteroids, offer symptomatic relief but do not result in definitive disease resolution. Surgery may be appropriate for certain patients, but recovery may be protracted and is associated with pain and discomfort. The ideal management should accomplish its goal in a short period of time with little discomfort or disability to the patient. Novel management methods should aim to stimulate a healing response to restore the normal biomechanical properties of tendon.

Cytokines and growth factors

The use of growth factors remains largely experimental and has been restricted to in vitro studies and animal models. The clinical use of growth factors for tendon problems has not been reported.

Insulin-like growth factor (IGF) is expressed in avian flexor tendons, and induces tenocyte migration, division, and matrix expression [50–52]. IGF-I and -II increase collagen synthesis in a dose-dependent manner in animal models, and also increase proteoglycan synthesis [50,53]. The response to cytokines may be site-specific; IGF-I induces a greater rate of collagen synthesis in rabbit flexor tendons compared with Achilles tendons [50].

IGF-I acts synergistically with platelet-derived growth factor (PDGF)-BB to stimulate tenocyte migration [50,51]. IGF-I and PDGF also act synergistically with cyclical loading and stimulate tenocytes mitogenically and matrigenically [54].

Intratendinous injection of IGF-1 was evaluated in a rat Achilles tendon transection model. Rats in the group that was treated with IGF-1 had higher Achilles functional index scores and accelerated recovery compared with control groups [55]. Degenerate equine flexor tendons that were injected locally with

IGF-I demonstrated decreased soft tissue swelling, increased DNA and collagen synthesis, improved echodensity of degenerate lesions, and improved tendon biomechanics compared with control tendons that were injected with saline [56].

Vascular endothelial growth factor (VEGF) is an endothelial mitogen that promotes angiogenesis and increases capillary permeability [57,58]. VEGF is expressed in ruptured and fetal human Achilles tendons, but not in normal adult Achilles tendons [59]. VEGF plays a key role in tendon healing. In a canine flexor tendon repair model, the expression of VEGF mRNA was increased at the repair site 7 days postoperatively, with peak levels occurring 10 days after surgery [60,61]. VEGF-induced vasodilatation results partly through stimulation of nitric oxide synthase in endothelial cells [62].

VEGF treatment at the time of surgical repair of transected rat Achilles tendons resulted in significantly improved tensile strength at 2 weeks, when the plantaris tendon was preserved [63]. No significant difference was present by 4 weeks.

Increased levels of transforming growth factor (TGF)-β2 have been reported in tendinopathic human Achilles tendons and in rabbit flexor tendons after injury [64,65]. TGF-β induces increased collagen production in rabbit tenocytes; up-regulation of TGF-β receptors occurs following flexor tendon injury and in tendinopathic human Achilles tendons [65–67]. TGF-β results in scar formation and fibrosis; TGF-β1 expression is increased in patients who have postburn hypertrophic scarring and keloids [68,69]. A single dose of antibody to TGF-β1 at the time of flexor tendon repair in rabbits produced an increased range of motion after surgery compared with control specimens [70].

Cartilage-derived morphogenetic proteins (CDMP), the human analogs of growth and differentiation factors (GDFs), are members of the TGF-β super-family, and are related to bone morphogenetic proteins [71]. Tendon tissue for-mation occurs when demineralized bone matrix that is coated with GDF-5, -6, and -7 is implanted into ectopic sites in rats [72]. Achilles tendons from GDF-5–deficient mice are weaker and contain less collagen than tendons from control mice [73]. Injection of CDMP-1, -2, and -3 into lacerated rat Achilles tendons resulted in a significant dose-related increase in strength and stiffness [74]. CDMP-2 injection into transected rabbit Achilles tendons resulted in a 35% increase in mechanical strength 14 days postoperatively compared with controls [75].

Not all cytokines prove beneficial for tendon healing. For example, tendinopathic equine flexor tendons that were treated with recombinant equine growth hormone had lower ultimate and yield tensile stress, with reduced stiff-ness [76]. Several issues need to be clarified before cytokine therapy becomes an established management modality. The ideal cytokine, or combination of cytokines, to improve tendon healing needs to be determined. Cytokine effects often are dose-dependent and optimal dosage regimes need to be established. The ideal form of administration also remains to be determined. Options include direct injection at the injury site or gene therapy [77]. Further research will help to resolve these issues.

In tendinopathy, a haphazard healing response occurs as a result of repetitive injury. Cytokine therapy may promote normal tendon healing, and therefore, has potential clinical application in tendinopathy. In addition, cytokine therapy could be used as a adjunct to surgical repair in cases of tendon rupture.

Gene therapy

Gene therapy delivers genetic material to cells to alter synthesis and function, and can be achieved by way of viral vectors or liposomes [78,79]. Several animal studies have investigated the feasibility of gene transfer to tendons. Liposome constructs have been used to deliver β-galactosidase to rat patellar tendons [80]. In vivo and ex vivo adenoviral transduction of the lac Z gene into rabbit patellar tenocytes has been reported. Gene expression lasted for 6 weeks, possibly long enough for clinical applications [81,82]. Apart from direct injection of vectors, gene transfer has been achieved by way of intra-arterial injection of liposomes [83].

Animal studies demonstrated that gene therapy can be used to alter the healing environment of tendons. Adenoviral transfection of focal adhesion kinase into partially lacerated chicken flexor tendons resulted in an expected increase in adhesion formation [84]. Although this study reported an adverse outcome, it proves the feasibility of gene therapy as a management modality.

Collagen type V plays a role in regulating the diameter of collagen type I during fibrillogenesis [85,86]. During healing, levels of collagen type V increase; persistently elevated levels have been found up to 52 weeks after injury in the rabbit medial collateral ligament. Elevated levels of collagen type V may favor the formation of smaller type I collagen fibrils, which, in turn, results in reduced mechanical strength [86,87]. Human patellar tenocytes that were transfected with specific antisense oligonucleotides synthesized reduced amounts of collagen type V [88].

Complementary DNA for PDGF-B was transfected into rat patellar tendons using liposomes [79]. The medial half of the patellar tendon was transected. PDGF-B resulted in an early increase in angiogenesis, and collagen deposition and matrix synthesis was greater at 4 weeks; however, there were no differences between the treated and control groups by 8 weeks.

Bone morphogenetic protein (BMP)-12 is the human analog of murine GDF-7 [89]. BMP-12 increases procollagen type I and III gene expression in human patellar tenocytes and is found at sites of tendon remodeling [90]. BMP-12 increased collagen type I synthesis by 30% in chicken flexor tenocytes; when tenocytes that were transfected with the BMP-12 gene were applied to a chicken flexor tendon laceration model, a two-fold increase in tensile strength and load to failure was seen after 4 weeks [91].

Gene therapy can be used to manipulate the healing environment for up to 8 to 10 weeks. This may be long enough to be clinically significant. Many genes may prove beneficial to tendon healing; further research is required to establish the most advantageous genes to transfer. The studies that were reviewed above have been conducted in tendon transection models, but gene therapy also may improve healing in tendinopathy.

Tissue engineering

Mesenchymal stem cells (MSCs) are capable of undergoing differentiation into a variety of specialized mesenchymal tissues, including bone, tendon, cartilage, muscle, ligament, fat, and marrow stroma [92]. In adults, MSCs are prevalent in bone marrow, but also are found in muscle, fat, skin, and around blood vessels [93].

MSCs can be applied directly to the site of injury or can be delivered on a suitable carrier matrix, which functions as a scaffold while tissue repair takes place. Muscle-derived progenitor cells that were injected into the supraspinatus tendon of nude rats differentiated into tenoblasts and became incorporated into collagen bundles [94]. Such a technique could be used to deliver autologous MSCs to areas of tendinopathy to stimulate healing.

Tissue engineering also may prove useful for managing tendon ruptures. A 1-cm long gap injury model in rabbit Achilles tendons was used to compare suture alone with a cell-collagen gel composite that was contracted onto a pre-tensioned suture [95]. Evaluation at 4, 8, and 12 weeks following surgery revealed that structural and material properties of the cell-treated implants typically were approximately twice the value of controls. Cell-treated repairs were larger in cross-section and better organized histologically than repairs that were done with suture alone.

Rabbit Achilles tendon defects that were treated with a core suture that was encapsulated in human amnion extracellular matrix seeded with fetal skin fibroblasts regained 81.8% of normal tensile strength after 3 months [96]. Window defects in rabbit patellar tendons were treated with autologous MSCs that were seeded onto a collagen implant, whereas unseeded collagen implants were placed into the control limb [97]. At 4 weeks, the MSC repairs had greater maximum stress (26%) and strain energy density (33%) than matched control.

Polyglycolic acid scaffolds that were seeded with tenocytes were implanted into hen flexor tendon defects [98]. Twelve weeks after surgery, tenocytes and collagen fibers became longitudinally aligned. At 14 weeks, engineered tendons displayed a typical tendon structure with a breaking strength of 83% of normal.

Another potential application of MSCs is ex vivo, de novo tissue engineering. This technique involves construction of whole body tissues in the laboratory, and their subsequent implantation into patients. Tissue-engineered tendons could be used to bridge areas of tissue loss or to replace severely tendinopathic regions.

Tissue engineering is an emerging field, and many difficulties need to be overcome before this becomes a real option in the management of tendon disorders. It is important to determine whether effective vascularization and innervation of implanted tissue-engineered constructs takes place. Vascularization is important for the viability of the construct. Innervation is required for proprioception and to maintain reflexes that are mediated by Golgi tendon organs to protect tendons from excessive forces [99,100].

Physical modalities

Several studies evaluated the application of electrical and magnetic fields to tendons. Pulsed magnetic fields with a frequency of 17 Hz resulted in improved collagen fiber alignment in a rat Achilles tendinopathy model [101]. Tenotomized rat Achilles tendons were sutured and treated with low-intensity galvanic current for 15 minutes a day for 2 weeks [102]. Biomechanical analysis revealed an increased force to breakage in the anode-stimulated group compared with controls and the cathode-stimulated group.

Extracorporeal shock wave therapy that was applied to rabbit Achilles tendons, at a rate of 500 impulses of 14 kV in 20 minutes, resulted in neovascularization and an increase in the angiogenesis-related markers, endothelial nitric oxide synthase and VEGF [103]. Extracorporeal shock wave therapy also promoted healing of Achilles tendinopathy in rats [104]. The investigators proposed that improvement in healing was a result of an increase in growth factor levels, because they noted elevated levels of TGF-β1 in the early stage and persistently elevated levels of IGF-1 [104]. Caution should be exercised when using extracorporeal shock wave therapy, however, because dose-dependent tendon damage, including fibrinoid necrosis, fibrosis, and inflammation, has been reported in rabbits [105].

Laser therapy also has been studied in tendon healing. In rabbits that were subjected to tenotomy and surgical repair of the Achilles tendon, laser phototherapy resulted in increased collagen production [106]. Using a placebo-controlled, double-blind prospective study model in 25 patients who had 41 digital flexor tendon repairs, laser therapy reduced postoperative edema, but no improvement in pain, grip strength, or functional evaluation was found compared with controls [107]. Further well-controlled clinical studies should be performed using different laser types and dosages to delineate the role of laser phototherapy in the management of tendon injuries.

Radiofrequency coblation is a new application of bipolar radiofrequency energy that is used for volumetric tissue removal. Under appropriate conditions, a small vapor layer forms on the active electrode of the device. The electrical field on the energized electrode causes electrical breakdown of the vapor; this produces a highly reactive plasma that is able to break down most of the bonds that are found in soft tissue molecules. Radiofrequency coblation stimulated an angiogenic response in normal rabbit Achilles tendons [108]. Rapid pain relief was reported in a preliminary prospective, nonrandomized, single-center, single-surgeon study of 20 patients who had tendinopathy of the Achilles tendon, patellar tendon, or the common extensor origin [108]. Six months after the procedure, MRI showed complete or near complete resolution of the tendinopathy lesion in 10 of the 20 patients who were enrolled in the study.

Physical modalities for the management of tendon disorders have been studied in animal models or small clinical trials. Despite being in clinical use, few controlled clinical trials have been performed; most of the evidence is preclinical, and, at times, controversial. Large-scale randomized controlled trials are required to establish clear guidelines on the indication and application of physical modalities.

Adhesion prevention

Trauma is the most important factor that is implicated in adhesion formation [109]. Many attempts have been made to reduce adhesion formation using materials that act as mechanical barriers (eg, polyethylene, silicone) or pharmacologic agents (eg, indomethacin, ibuprofen) however; no simple method is used widely [110–113].

Hyaluronate, a high molecular weight polysaccharide that is found in synovial fluid around tendon sheaths, decreased adhesion formation in rabbit flexor tendons [114,115]; however, no statistically significant difference in adhesion formation was found in a rat Achilles tendon model [116]. The absence of a synovial membrane around the Achilles tendon may explain this difference. 5-Fluorouracil, an antimetabolite with anti-inflammatory properties, effectively preserved tendon gliding in lacerated chicken flexor tendons [117–119].

Physical modalities also have been used in an attempt to limit adhesion formation. Direct current that was applied to rabbit tendons in vitro resulted in increased collagen type I production and reduced adhesion formation [120]; however, pulsed electromagnetic field stimulation resulted in no difference in adhesion formation in rabbit flexor tendons after 4 weeks [121].

Despite many efforts, adhesion formation after trauma to tendons remains a clinical problem, and no ideal method of prevention exists. Most studies on adhesion formation focus on flexor tendons. Further research is required to determine whether the results are also applicable to extrasynovial tendons.

Mobilization and mechanical loading

Animal experiments have demonstrated that training results in improved tensile strength, elastic stiffness, weight, and cross-sectional area of tendons [122,123]. These effects can be explained by an increase in collagen and extracellular matrix synthesis by tenocytes [123]. Little data exist on the effect of exercise on human tendons, although intensively-trained athletes are reported to have thicker Achilles tendons than control subjects [124].

Prolonged immobilization following musculoskeletal injury may result in detrimental effects. Collagen fascicles from stress-shielded rabbit patellar tendons displayed reduced tensile strength and strain at failure than control samples [125]. Immobilization reduces the water and proteoglycan content of tendons, and increases the number of reducible collagen cross-links [126,127].

Early resumption of activity promotes restoration of function; motion therapy strategies aim to facilitate healing, reduce adhesion formation, and increase range of motion [128,129]. Many studies showed the benefit of early mobilization following tendon repair, and several postoperative mobilization protocols have been advocated [130–132]. Repetitive motion results in increased DNA content and protein synthesis in human tenocytes [133]. Even 15 minutes of cyclic biaxial mechanical strain that is applied to human tenocytes results in cellular proliferation [134]. Application of cyclic load to wounded avian flexor tendons resulted in epitenon cell migration into the wound [135]. In rabbit patellar tendons, application of a 4% strain provided protection against degradation by bacterial collagenase [136].

The precise mechanism by which cells respond to load remains to be elucidated; however, cells must respond to mechanical and chemical signals in a coordinated fashion. Intercellular communication, to mount mitogenic and matrigenic responses, is achieved by way of gap junctions ex vivo [54]. Tissue-engineered tendons must allow for this intercellular communication. Mechanical loading of cells in monolayer or three-dimensional constructs can result in increased cell proliferation and collagen synthesis [137].

Summary

Tendon injuries give rise to significant morbidity, and, at present, only limited scientifically-proven management modalities exist. A better understanding of tendon function and healing will allow specific management strategies to be developed. Many interesting techniques are being pioneered. The optimization strategies that were discussed in this article are at an early stage of development. Although these emerging technologies may develop into substantial clinical management options, their full impact needs to be evaluated critically in a scientific fashion.

References

[1] Kirkendall DT, Garrett WE. Function and biomechanics of tendons. Scand J Med Sci Sports 1997;7(2):62–6.

[2] O'Brien M. Functional anatomy and physiology of tendons. Clin Sports Med 1992;11:505–20.

[3] Oxlund H. Relationships between the biomechanical properties, composition and molecular structure of connective tissues. Connect Tissue Res 1986;15(1–2):65–72.

[4] Carlstedt CA, Nordin M. Biomechanics of tendons and ligaments. In: Nordin M, Frankel VH, editors. Basic biomechanics of the musculoskeletal system. Philadelphia: Lea and Ferbiger; 1989. p. 59–74.

[5] Viidik A. Tendons and ligaments. In: Comper W, editor. Extracellular matrix, vol. 1. Amsterdam: Harwood Academic Publishers; 1996. p. 303–27.

[6] Fyfe I, Stanish WD. The use of eccentric training and stretching in the treatment and prevention of tendon injuries. Clin Sports Med 1992;11(3):601–24.

[7] Zernicke RF, Loitz BJ. Exercise-related adaptations in connective tissue. In: Komi PV, editor. The encyclopaedia of sports medicine. Strength and power in sport. Oxford (UK): Blackwell; 2002. p. 93–113.

[8] Mosler E, Folkhard W, Knorzer E, et al. Stress-induced molecular rearrangement in tendon collagen. J Mol Biol 1985;182(4):589–96.

[9] Curwin SL, Stanish WD. Tendinitis: its etiology and treatment. Lexington (MA): Collamore Press; 1984.

[10] Butler DL, Grood ES, Noyes FR, et al. Biomechanics of ligaments and tendons. Exerc Sport Sci Rev 1978;6:125–81.

[11] Kastelic J, Baer E. Deformation in tendon collagen. Symp Soc Exp Biol 1980;34:397–435.

[12] Elliot D. Structure and function of mammalian tendon. Biol Rev 1965;40:392–421.

[13] Shadwick RE. Elastic energy storage in tendons: mechanical differences related to function and age. J Appl Physiol 1990;68(3):1033–40.

[14] Komi PV, Salonen M, Jarvinen M, et al. In vivo registration of Achilles tendon forces in man. I. Methodological development. Int J Sports Med 1987;8(Suppl 1):3–8.

[15] Komi PV. Relevance of in vivo force measurements to human biomechanics. J Biomech 1990;23(Suppl 1):23–34.

[16] Komi PV, Fukashiro S, Jarvinen M. Biomechanical loading of Achilles tendon during normal locomotion. Clin Sports Med 1992;11(3):521–31.

[17] Leadbetter WB. Cell-matrix response in tendon injury. Clin Sports Med 1992;11(3):533–78.

[18] Frank CB, Bray RC, Hart DA, et al. Soft tissue healing. In: Fu F, Harner CD, Vince KG, editors. Knee surgery. Baltimore (MD): Williams and Wilkins; 1994. p. 189–224.

[19] Murphy PG, Loitz BJ, Frank CB, et al. Influence of exogenous growth factors on the synthesis and secretion of collagen types I and III by explants of normal and healing rabbit ligaments. Biochem Cell Biol 1994;72:403–9.

[20] Oakes BW. Tissue healing and repair: tendons and ligaments. In: Frontera WR, editor. Rehabilitation of sports injuries: scientific basis. Oxford (UK): Blackwell Science; 2003. p. 56–98.

[21] Tillman LJ, Chasan NP. Properties of dense connective tissue and wound healing. In: Hertling RM, Kessler RM, editors. Management of common musculoskeletal disorders. Philadelphia: Lippincott; 1996. p. 8–20.

[22] Hooley CJ, Cohen RE. A model for the creep behaviour of tendon. Int J Biol Macromol 1979; 1:123–32.

[23] Akeson WH, Woo SL, Amiel D, et al. Immobility effects on synovial joints. The pathomechanics of joint contractures. Biorheology 1980;17:95–110.

[24] Abrahamsson SO. Matrix metabolism and healing in the flexor tendon. Experimental studies on rabbit tendon. Scand J Plast Reconstr Surg Hand Surg Suppl 1991;23:1–51.

[25] Farkas LG, McCain WG, Sweeney P, et al. An experimental study of changes following silastic rod preparation of new tendon sheath and subsequent tendon grafting. J Bone Joint Surg Am 1973;55(6):149–58.

[26] Madden JW, Peacock EE. Studies on the biology of collagen during wound healing III: dynamic metabolism of scar collagen and remodeling of dermal wounds. Ann Surg 1971;174: 511–20.

[27] Amiel D, Akeson W, Harwood FL, et al. Stress deprivation effect on metabolic turnover of medial collateral ligament collagen. Clin Orthop 1987;172:25–7.

[28] Gelberman RH, Amiel D, Harwood F. Genetic expression for type I procollagen in the early stages of flexor tendon healing. J Hand Surg [Am] 1992;17:551–8.

[29] Garner WL, McDonald JA, Kuhn III C, et al. Autonomous healing of chicken flexor tendons in vitro. J Hand Surg [Am] 1988;13:697–700.

[30] Manske PR, Gelberman RH, Lesker PA. Flexor tendon healing. Hand Clin 1985;1(1):25–34.

[31] Gelberman RH, Manske PR, Akeson WH, et al. Flexor tendon repair. J Orthop Res 1986;4(1): 119–28.

[32] Tokita Y, Yamaya A, Yabe Y. [An experimental study on the repair and restoration of gliding function after digital flexor tendon injury. I. Repair of the sutured digital flexor tendon within digital sheath]. Nippon Seikeigeka Gakkai Zasshi [JP] 1974;48:107–27.

[33] Fujita M, Hukuda S, Doida Y. [Experimental study of intrinsic healing of the flexor tendon: collagen synthesis of the cultured flexor tendon cells of the canine]. Nippon Seikeigeka Gakkai Zasshi [JP] 1992;66(4):326–33.

[34] Ingraham JM, Hauck RM, Ehrlich HP. Is the tendon embryogenesis process resurrected during tendon healing? Plast Reconstr Surg 2003;112(3):844–54.

[35] Lundborg G, Rank F. Experimental studies on cellular mechanisms involved in healing of animal and human flexor tendon in synovial environment. Hand 1980;12(1):3–11.

[36] Lundborg G, Hansson HA, Rank F, et al. Superficial repair of severed flexor tendons in synovial environment. An experimental, ultrastructural study on cellular mechanisms. J Hand Surg [Am] 1980;5(5):451–61.

[37] Russell JE, Manske PR. Collagen synthesis during primate flexor tendon repair in vitro. J Orthop Res 1990;8(1):13–20.

[38] Becker H, Graham MF, Cohen IK, et al. Intrinsic tendon cell proliferation in tissue culture. J Hand Surg [Am] 1981;6(6):616–9.

[39] Koob TJ. Biomimetic approaches to tendon repair. Comp Biochem Physiol A Mol Integr Physiol 2002;133(4):1171–92.

[40] Koob TJ, Summers AP. Tendon-bridging the gap. Comp Biochem Physiol A Mol Integr Physiol 2002;133(4):905–9.

[41] Strickland JW. Flexor tendons: acute injuries. In: Green D, Hotchkiss R, Pedersen W, editors. Green's operative hand surgery. New York: Churchill Livingstone; 1999. p. 1851–97.

[42] Uhthoff HK, Sarkar K. Surgical repair of rotator cuff ruptures. The importance of the subacromial bursa. J Bone Joint Surg Br 1991;73(3):399–401.

[43] Evans CH. Cytokines and the role they play in the healing of ligaments and tendons. Sports Med 1999;28(2):71–6.

[44] Sciore P, Boykiw R, Hart DA. Semiquantitative reverse transcription-polymerase chain reaction analysis of mRNA for growth factors and growth factor receptors from normal and healing rabbit medial collateral ligament tissue. J Orthop Res 1998;16:429–37.

[45] Chang J, Most D, Stelnicki E, et al. Gene expression of transforming growth factor beta-1 in rabbit zone II flexor tendon wound healing: evidence for dual mechanisms of repair. Plast Reconstr Surg 1997;100(4):937–44.

[46] Chang J, Most D, Thunder R, et al. Molecular studies in flexor tendon wound healing: the role of basic fibroblast growth factor gene expression. J Hand Surg [Am] 1998;23A:1052–8.

[47] Woo SL, Hildebrand K, Watanabe N, et al. Tissue engineering of ligaments and tendon healing. Clin Orthop 1999;367:S312–23.

[48] Natsu-ume T, Nakamura N, Shino K, et al. Temporal and spatial expression of transforming growth factor–beta in the healing patellar ligament of the rat. J Orthop Res 1997;15(6):837–43.

[49] Marui T, Niyibizi C, Georgescu HI, et al. Effect of growth factors on matrix synthesis by ligament fibroblasts. J Orthop Res 1997;15(1):18–23.

[50] Abrahamsson SO, Lohmander S. Differential effects of insulin-like growth factor-I on matrix and DNA synthesis in various regions and types of rabbit tendons. J Orthop Res 1996;14(3): 370–6.

[51] Banes AJ, Tsuzaki M, Hu P, et al. PDGF-BB, IGF-I and mechanical load stimulate DNA synthesis in avian tendon fibroblasts in vitro. J Biomech 1995;28:1505–13.

[52] Tsuzaki M, Xiao H, Brigman B, et al. IGF-I is expressed by avian flexor tendon cells. J Orthop Res 2000;8:546–56.

[53] Murphy DJ, Nixon AJ. Biochemical and site-specific effects of insulin-like growth factor I on intrinsic tenocyte activity in equine flexor tendons. Am J Vet Res 1997;58(1):103–9.

[54] Banes AJ, Horesovsky G, Larson C, et al. Mechanical load stimulates expression of novel genes in vivo and in vitro in avian flexor tendon cells. Osteoarthritis Cartilage 1999;7:141–53.

[55] Kurtz CA, Loebig TG, Anderson DD, et al. Insulin-like growth factor I accelerates functional recovery from Achilles tendon injury in a rat model. Am J Sports Med 1999;27(3):363–9.

[56] Dahlgren LA, van der Meulen MC, Bertram JE, et al. Insulin-like growth factor-I improves cellular and molecular aspects of healing in a collagenase-induced model of flexor tendinitis. J Orthop Res 2002;20(5):910–9.

[57] Ferrara N. Role of vascular endothelial growth factor in the regulation of angiogenesis. Kidney Int 1999;56(3):794–814.

[58] Neufeld G, Cohen T, Gengrinovitch S, et al. Vascular endothelial growth factor (VEGF) and its receptors. FASEB J 1999;13(1):9–22.

[59] Pufe T, Petersen W, Tillmann B, et al. The angiogenic peptide vascular endothelial growth factor is expressed in foetal and ruptured tendons. Virchows Arch 2001;439(4):579–85.

[60] Bidder M, Towler DA, Gelberman RH, et al. Expression of mRNA for vascular endothelial growth factor at the repair site of healing canine flexor tendon. J Orthop Res 2000;18(2): 247–52.

[61] Boyer MI, Watson JT, Lou J, et al. Quantitative variation in vascular endothelial growth factor mRNA expression during early flexor tendon healing: an investigation in a canine model. J Orthop Res 2001;19(5):869–72.

[62] Yang R, Thomas GR, Bunting S, et al. Effects of vascular endothelial growth factor on hemodynamics and cardiac performance. J Cardiovasc Pharmacol 1996;27(6):838–44.

[63] Zhang F, Liu H, Stile F, et al. Effect of vascular endothelial growth factor on rat Achilles tendon healing. Plast Reconstr Surg 2003;112(6):1613–9.

[64] Chang J, Most D, Stelnicki E, et al. Gene expression of transforming growth factor beta–1 in rabbit zone II flexor tendon wound healing: evidence for dual mechanisms of repair. Plast Reconstr Surg 1997;100(4):937–44.

[65] Fenwick SA, Curry V, Harrall RL, et al. Expression of transforming growth factor-beta isoforms and their receptors in chronic tendinosis. J Anat 2001;199(Pt 3):231–40.

[66] Klein MB, Yalamanchi N, Pham H, et al. Flexor tendon healing in vitro: effects of TGF-beta on tendon cell collagen production. J Hand Surg [Am] 2002;27(4):615–20.

[67] Ngo M, Pham H, Longaker MT, et al. Differential expression of transforming growth factor-beta receptors in a rabbit zone II flexor tendon wound healing model. Plast Reconstr Surg 2001;108(5):1260–7.

[68] Ghahary A, Shen YJ, Scott PG, et al. Enhanced expression of mRNA for transforming growth factor-beta, type I and type III procollagen in human post-burn hypertrophic scar tissues. J Lab Clin Med 1993;122(4):465–73.

[69] Peltonen J, Hsiao LL, Jaakkola S, et al. Activation of collagen gene expression in keloids: co-localization of type I and VI collagen and transforming growth factor-beta 1 mRNA. J Invest Dermatol 1991;97(2):240–8.

[70] Chang J, Thunder R, Most D, et al. Studies in flexor tendon wound healing: neutralizing antibody to TGF-beta1 increases postoperative range of motion. Plast Reconstr Surg 2000; 105(1):148–55.

[71] Chang SC, Hoang B, Thomas JT, et al. Cartilage-derived morphogenetic proteins. New members of the transforming growth factor-beta superfamily predominantly expressed in long bones during human embryonic development. J Biol Chem 1994;269(45):28227–34.

[72] Wolfman NM, Hattersley G, Cox K, et al. Ectopic induction of tendon and ligament in rats by growth and differentiation factors 5, 6, and 7, members of the TGF-beta gene family. J Clin Invest 1997;100(2):321–30.

[73] Mikic B, Schalet BJ, Clark RT, et al. GDF-5 deficiency in mice alters the ultrastructure, mechanical properties and composition of the Achilles tendon. J Orthop Res 2001;19(3):365–71.

[74] Forslund C, Rueger D, Aspenberg P. A comparative dose-response study of cartilage-derived morphogenetic protein (CDMP)-1, -2 and -3 for tendon healing in rats. J Orthop Res 2003; 21(4):617–21.

[75] Forslund C, Aspenberg P. Improved healing of transected rabbit Achilles tendon after a single injection of cartilage-derived morphogenetic protein-2. Am J Sports Med 2003;31(4):555–9.

[76] Dowling BA, Dart AJ, Hodgson DR, et al. Recombinant equine growth hormone does not affect the in vitro biomechanical properties of equine superficial digital flexor tendon. Vet Surg 2002;31(4):325–30.

[77] Muzzonigro TS, Ghivizzani SC, Robbins PD, et al. The role of gene therapy. Fact or fiction? Clin Sports Med 1999;18(1):223–39.

[78] Nakamura N, Timmermann SA, Hart DA, et al. A comparison of in vivo gene delivery methods for antisense therapy in ligament healing. Gene Ther 1998;5(11):1455–61.

[79] Nakamura N, Shino K, Natsuume T, et al. Early biological effect of in vivo gene transfer of platelet-derived growth factor (PDGF)-B into healing patellar ligament. Gene Ther 1998;5(9):1165–70.

[80] Nakamura N, Horibe S, Matsumoto N, et al. Transient introduction of a foreign gene into healing rat patellar ligament. J Clin Invest 1996;97(1):226–31.

[81] Gerich TG, Kang R, Fu FH, et al. Gene transfer to the rabbit patellar tendon: potential for genetic enhancement of tendon and ligament healing. Gene Ther 1996;3(12):1089–93.

[82] Gerich TG, Kang R, Fu FH, et al. Gene transfer to the patellar tendon. Knee Surg Sports Traumatol Arthrosc 1997;5(2):118–23.

[83] Ozkan I, Shino K, Nakamura N, et al. Direct in vivo gene transfer to healing rat patellar ligament by intra-arterial delivery of haemagglutinating virus of Japan liposomes. Eur J Clin Invest 1999;29(1):63–7.

[84] Lou J, Kubota H, Hotokezaka S, et al. In vivo gene transfer and overexpression of focal adhesion kinase (pp125 FAK) mediated by recombinant adenovirus-induced tendon adhesion formation and epitenon cell change. J Orthop Res 1997;15(6):911–8.

[85] Marchant JK, Hahn RA, Linsenmayer TF, et al. Reduction of type V collagen using a dominant-negative strategy alters the regulation of fibrillogenesis and results in the loss of corneal-specific fibril morphology. J Cell Biol 1996;135(5):1415–26.

[86] Adachi E, Hayashi T. In vitro formation of hybrid fibrils of type V collagen and type I collagen. Limited growth of type I collagen into thick fibrils by type V collagen. Connect Tissue Res 1986;14(4):257–66.

[87] Niyibizi C, Kavalkovich K, Yamaji T, et al. Type V collagen is increased during rabbit medial collateral ligament healing. Knee Surg Sports Traumatol Arthrosc 2000;8:281–5.

[88] Shimomura T, Jia F, Niyibizi C, et al. Antisense oligonucleotides reduce synthesis of procollagen alpha1 (V) chain in human patellar tendon fibroblasts: potential application in healing ligaments and tendons. Connect Tissue Res 2003;44(3–4):167–72.

[89] Wolfman NM, Celeste AJ, Cox K, et al. Preliminary characterization of the biological activities of rhBMP-12. J Bone Miner Res 1995;10:s148–54.

[90] Fu SC, Wong YP, Chan BP, et al. The roles of bone morphogenetic protein (BMP) 12 in stimulating the proliferation and matrix production of human patellar tendon fibroblasts. Life Sci 2003;72(26):2965–74.

[91] Lou J, Tu Y, Burns M, et al. BMP-12 gene transfer augmentation of lacerated tendon repair. J Orthop Res 2001;19:1199–202.

[92] Caplan AI. The mesengenic process. Clin Plast Surg 1994;21(3):429–35.

[93] Caplan AI, Bruder SP. Mesenchymal stem cells: building blocks for molecular medicine in the 21st century. Trends Mol Med 2001;7(6):259–64.

[94] Pelinkovic D, Lee JY, Engelhardt M, et al. Muscle cell-mediated gene delivery to the rotator cuff. Tissue Eng 2003;9(1):143–51.

[95] Young RG, Butler DL, Weber W, et al. Use of mesenchymal stem cells in a collagen matrix for Achilles tendon repair. J Orthop Res 1998;16(4):406–13.

[96] He Q, Li Q, Chen B, et al. Repair of flexor tendon defects of rabbit with tissue engineering method. Chin J Traumatol 2002;5(4):200–8.

[97] Awad HA, Butler DL, Boivin GP, et al. Autologous mesenchymal stem cell-mediated repair of tendon. Tissue Eng 1999;5(3):267–77.

[98] Cao Y, Liu Y, Liu W, et al. Bridging tendon defects using autologous tenocyte engineered tendon in a hen model. Plast Reconstr Surg 2002;110(5):1280–9.

 [99] Powers S, Howley E. Exercise physiology: theory and application to fitness and performance. New York: McGraw-Hill; 2001.
[100] Baechle T, Earle R. Essentials of strength training and conditioning. Champaign (IL): Human Kinetics; 2000.
[101] Lee EW, Maffulli N, Li CK, et al. Pulsed magnetic and electromagnetic fields in experimental Achilles tendonitis in the rat: a prospective randomized study. Arch Phys Med Rehab 1997;78(4):399–404.
[102] Owoeye I, Spielholz NI, Fetto J, et al. Low-intensity pulsed galvanic current and the healing of tenotomized rat Achilles tendons: preliminary report using load-to-breaking measurements. Arch Phys Med Rehabil 1987;68(7):415–8.
[103] Wang CJ, Wang FS, Yang KD, et al. Shock wave therapy induces neovascularization at the tendon-bone junction. A study in rabbits. J Orthop Res 2003;21(6):984–9.
[104] Chen YJ, Wang CJ, Yang KD, et al. Extracorporeal shock waves promote healing of collagenase-induced Achilles tendinitis and increase TGF-beta1 and IGF-I expression. J Orthop Res 2004;22(4):854–61.
[105] Rompe JD, Kirkpatrick CJ, Kullmer K, et al. Dose-related effects of shock waves on rabbit tendo Achilles. A sonographic and histological study. J Bone Joint Surg Br 1998;80(3): 546–52.
[106] Reddy GK, Stehno-Bittel L, Enwemeka CS. Laser photostimulation of collagen production in healing rabbit Achilles tendons. Lasers Surg Med 1998;22(5):281–7.
[107] Ozkan N, Altan L, Bingol U, et al. Investigation of the supplementary effect of GaAs laser therapy on the rehabilitation of human digital flexor tendons. J Clin Laser Med Surg 2004;22(2):105–10.
[108] Tasto JP, Cummings J, Medlock V, et al. The tendon treatment center: new horizons in the treatment of tendinosis. Arthroscopy 2003;19(Suppl 1):213–23.
[109] Jaibaji M. Advances in the biology of zone II flexor tendon healing and adhesion formation. Ann Plast Surg 2000;45(1):83–92.
[110] Hunter JM, Salisbury RE. Flexor-tendon reconstruction in severely damaged hands. A two-stage procedure using a silicone-dacron reinforced gliding prosthesis prior to tendon grafting. J Bone Joint S Am 1971;53(5):829–58.
[111] Nishimura K, Nakamura RM, diZerega GS. Ibuprofen inhibition of postsurgical adhesion formation: a time and dose response biochemical evaluation in rabbits. J Surg Res 1984;36(2): 115–24.
[112] Nishimura K, Shimanuki T, diZerega GS. Ibuprofen in the prevention of experimentally induced postoperative adhesions. Am J Med 1984;77(1A):102–6.
[113] Szabo RM, Younger E. Effects of indomethacin on adhesion formation after repair of zone II tendon lacerations in the rabbit. J Hand Surg [Am] 1990;15(3):480–3.
[114] Hagberg L, Heinegard D, Ohlsson K. The contents of macromolecule solutes in flexor tendon sheath fluid and their relation to synovial fluid. A quantitative analysis. J Hand Surg [Br] 1992; 17(2):167–71.
[115] Hagberg L, Gerdin B. Sodium hyaluronate as an adjunct in adhesion prevention after flexor tendon surgery in rabbits. J Hand Surg [Am] 1992;17(5):935–41.
[116] Tuncay I, Ozbek H, Atik B, et al. Effects of hyaluronic acid on postoperative adhesion of tendo calcaneus surgery: an experimental study in rats. J Foot Ankle Surg 2002;41(2):104–8.
[117] Khan U, Occleston NL, Khaw PT, et al. Single exposures to 5-fluorouracil: a possible mode of targeted therapy to reduce contractile scarring in the injured tendon. Plast Reconstr Surg 1997; 99(2):465–71.
[118] Khan U, Kakar S, Akali A, et al. Modulation of the formation of adhesions during the healing of injured tendons. J Bone Joint Surg Br 2000;82(7):1054–8.
[119] Moran SL, Ryan CK, Orlando GS, et al. Effects of 5-fluorouracil on flexor tendon repair. J Hand Surg [Am] 2000;25(2):242–51.
[120] Fujita M, Hukuda S, Doida Y. The effect of constant direct electrical current on intrinsic healing in the flexor tendon in vitro. An ultrastructural study of differing attitudes in epitenon cells and tenocytes. J Hand Surg [Br] 1992;17(1):94–8.

[121] Greenough CG. The effect of pulsed electromagnetic fields on flexor tendon healing in the rabbit. J Hand Surg [Br] 1996;21(6):808–12.

[122] Kannus P, Józsa KP, Renstrom P, et al. The effects of training, immobilization and remobilization on musculoskeletal tissue: 1: training and immobilization. Scan J Med Sci Sports 1992;2:100–18.

[123] Kannus P, Jozsa L, Natri A, et al. Effects of training, immobilization and remobilization on tendons. Scand J Med Sci Sports 1997;7(2):67–71.

[124] Maffulli N, King JB. Effects of physical activity on some components of the skeletal system. Sports Med 1992;13(6):393–407.

[125] Yamamoto E, Hayashi K, Yamamoto N. Mechanical properties of collagen fascicles from stress-shielded patellar tendons in the rabbit. Clin Biomech 1999;14(6):418–25.

[126] Akeson WH, Woo SL, Amiel D, et al. The connective tissue response to immobility: biochemical changes in periarticular connective tissue of the immobilized rabbit knee. Clin Orthop 1973;93:356–62.

[127] Akeson WH, Amiel D, Mechanic GL, et al. Collagen cross-linking alterations in joint contractures: changes in the reducible cross-links in periarticular connective tissue collagen after nine weeks of immobilization. Connect Tissue Res 1977;5(1):15–9.

[128] Buckwalter JA. Activity vs. rest in the treatment of bone, soft tissue and joint injuries. Iowa Orthop J 1995;15:29–42.

[129] Buckwalter JA. Effects of early motion on healing of musculoskeletal tissues. Hand Clin 1996; 12(1):13–24.

[130] Chow JA, Thomes LJ, Dovelle S, et al. Controlled motion rehabilitation after flexor tendon repair and grafting. A multi-centre study. J Bone Joint Surg Br 1988;70(4):591–5.

[131] Cullen KW, Tolhurst P, Lang D, et al. Flexor tendon repair in zone 2 followed by controlled active mobilisation. J Hand Surg [Br] 1989;14(4):392–5.

[132] Elliot D, Moiemen NS, Flemming AF, et al. The rupture rate of acute flexor tendon repairs mobilized by the controlled active motion regimen. J Hand Surg [Br] 1994;19(5):607–12.

[133] Almekinders LC, Baynes AJ, Bracey LW. An in vitro investigation into the effects of repetitive motion and nonsteroidal antiinflammatory medication on human tendon fibroblasts. Am J Sports Med 1995;23(1):119–23.

[134] Zeichen J, van Griensven M, Bosch U. The proliferative response of isolated human tendon fibroblasts to cyclic biaxial mechanical strain. Am J Sports Med 2000;28(6):888–92.

[135] Tanaka H, Manske PR, Pruitt DL, et al. Effect of cyclic tension on lacerated flexor tendons in vitro. J Hand Surg [Am] 1995;20(3):467–73.

[136] Nabeshima Y, Grood ES, Sakurai A, et al. Uniaxial tension inhibits tendon collagen degradation by collagenase in vitro. J Orthop Res 1996;14(1):123–30.

[137] Banes AJ, Tsuzaki M, Yamamoto J, et al. Mechanoreception at the cellular level: the detection, interpretation, and diversity of responses to mechanical signals. Biochem Cell Biol 1995;73: 349–65.

ELSEVIER
SAUNDERS

Foot Ankle Clin N Am
10 (2005) 399–412

FOOT AND
ANKLE CLINICS

Index

Note: Page numbers of article titles are in **boldface** type.